We would like to dedicate this book to the men and women with esophageal cancer, along with their families, that we have had the opportunity to care for during their evaluation, treatment, and recovery. We have learned a tremendous amount from their strength and courage. They, along with the thousands of people diagnosed each year with cancer of the esophagus, inspire us and others to work toward improved education, treatment, and support for this disease.

Pamela K. Ginex, EdD, RN, OCN
Maureen Jingeleski, RN, BSN
Manjit S. Bains, MD

I would like to dedicate this book to Dominic A. Carone, who, in the short time I knew him, became a friend, a confidant, and a major contributor and partner in the creation of The Esophageal Cancer Education Foundation.

Dominic was instrumental in putting our Web site together, *www.fightec.org*, and with his passing in October of 2003, I not only lost a good friend but also lost a crusader who was strong in getting the message to the public, which is what we hope this book will do.

Bart L. Frazzitta

The diagnosis of esophageal cancer brings extraordinary emotional, physical, and practical challenges to both patients and those close to them. These challenges can seem overwhelming at times, but they are not insurmountable. We believe that knowledge is key to navigating a complex healthcare system and taking an active role in your care. In this book, *100 Questions & Answers About Esophageal Cancer, Second Edition*, our goal was to provide information that will help you to ask appropriate questions and be an effective patient. Our intention is to answer general questions about the disease, discuss treatment options, identify sources of support, and assist you in managing the side effects of the disease and treatment. Ideally, this information will help you and your loved ones know which questions to ask your doctors to make better informed decisions about your care. We hope that you find this book helpful.

Our inspiration for this book has been our remarkable patients. When faced with this difficult disease, they have shown us the true meaning of strength and courage. We are honored and privileged to care for them and continue to fight to improve treatments and outcomes. For the insight to see the enormous need for this book, we would like to thank Christopher Davis, Executive Publisher for Medicine at Jones and Bartlett Publishers. Esophageal cancer is not a cancer you hear about often, and Chris had the vision to see the need for this book. We also thank Terry Helms, medical illustrator at Memorial Sloan-Kettering, for her artistic illustrations. We would like to especially thank Jacqueline Hanson, RN, BSN, OCN, for her work on the first edition of this book and for her over 40 years of expert care and dedication to patients battling cancer. Her expertise and professionalism were an inspiration to us and a comfort to her patients.

Pamela K. Ginex, EdD, RN, OCN
Maureen Jingeleski, RN, BSN
Manjit S. Bains, MD

From a patient's perspective, it is important to get quality information about such an important topic as cancer in general, and esophageal cancer specifically. We certainly have the Internet and all of the information that it can provide, some of which is inaccurate, some of which is outdated, and some of which may be good.

To have a book that specifically addresses esophageal cancer and answers many of the questions one would have about this disease will provide a great comfort to the individual who has been informed that he or she has this disease. As a patient myself, when I first heard that I had esophageal cancer, I decided to not surf the Internet. However, my daughters did that for me, and all of the information that was by a consensus accurate, or at least seemed to be accurate, they shared with me. To have had a book about esophageal cancer that was written by leaders in this field at a time when we were gathering information about this disease would have provided a comfort level that would have made the process a lot easier and less tense.

I applaud the publishers and my coauthors of this book for the time and effort they have put into this task, and they should be proud of the resource they have placed before us. From my patient perspective, I cannot help but acknowledge the Memorial Sloan-Kettering doctors and nurses who have allowed me to be here today. Without the expertise and dedication that they bring to the patients in their care, cancer would be as dark a word as it was 10 to 20 years ago.

Through their efforts, more of us are living a quality of life that is somewhat comparable to that of our peers, and with the grace of God they will continue this quest and, hopefully, in our lifetime find a cure for this dreaded disease.

God bless us all.

Bart L. Frazzitta

PART ONE

The Basics

What is the esophagus?

What is cancer of the esophagus?

What causes esophageal cancer?

More . . .

Esophagus

A portion of the digestive canal, shaped like a hollow tube, which connects the throat to the stomach. Controlled muscle contractions propel food and liquids into the stomach, and muscles at the stomach form a valve (esophageal sphincter) that prevents the stomach contents from coming back up into the esophagus.

Gastroesophageal reflux disease (GERD)

A syndrome due to a structural or functional inability of the lower esophageal sphincter to prevent gastric juice from flooding back into the esophagus.

Esophagitis

Irritation, inflammation, or damage of the esophagus caused by regurgitation of the acid gastric contents.

Barrett's esophagus

A chronic ulceration of the lower esophagus from esophagitis or esophageal cancer that causes the normal lining to be replaced by cells similar to the stomach or intestine, which can tolerate the acid or bile without damage.

1. What is the esophagus?

The **esophagus** is a hollow, muscular tube about 10 inches long that connects the throat with the stomach. It lies in front and slightly to the right side of the spine behind the windpipe in the upper part of the chest, and behind the heart in the lower part of the chest.

2. What does the esophagus do?

There are several layers of muscle in the wall of the esophagus that, by coordinated contractions, help propel food and liquids into the stomach. At the junction where the esophagus meets the stomach, the muscle layers function as a valve to prevent any food from going back (refluxing) into the esophagus. All of us are prone to getting occasional episodes where the stomach contents, including food, acid, or bile, will reflux back into the esophagus. This causes "heartburn." Some people have reflux or heartburn frequently, and this is referred to as **gastroesophageal reflux disease** or **GERD** (see Question 12). Over time, frequent episodes of the esophageal lining being exposed to stomach acid or bile will cause damage to the normal lining of the esophagus. This damage is called **esophagitis**. Sometimes, after prolonged exposure to acid or bile, the normal lining is replaced by stomach or intestinal lining that can tolerate the acid or the bile without getting damaged or injured. This change in the lining of the esophagus is referred to as **Barrett's esophagus**. Chances of developing a cancer are significantly higher in the Barrett's esophageal lining than the normal (squamous) lining of the esophagus. **Figure 1** is an illustration of the esophagus in relation to other parts of the body.

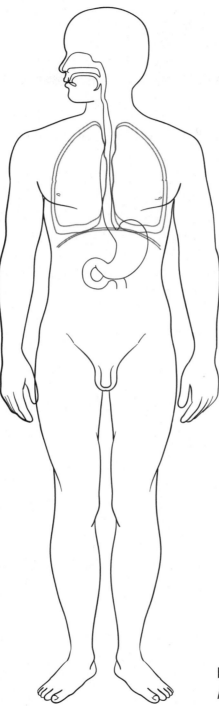

Figure 1
Anatomy of the chest.

3. What is cancer?

Cancer is the word used to describe a group of diseases that affect **cells** in our bodies. There are more than 100 types of cancer. In order to understand cancer, it is important to know how our cells normally function and the process that may lead to the development of cancer.

Normal Cells

Our bodies are made up of many different types of cells, with each type uniquely distinguishable from another. For example, a lung cell looks and acts very different from a stomach cell or a pancreatic cell. Each cell has a specific function to help keep us healthy and functioning properly. For example, red blood cells carry oxygen throughout the body and white blood cells help to fight infections. Cells each have a specific "lifespan" and will normally mature over a period of time and then stop growing. Red blood cells normally survive approximately 120 days before they are replaced by new red blood cells. Our bodies are continually at work producing more cells for when we need them. For example, if you have an infected cut on your finger, your body will produce more white blood cells to fight off the infection; then, when the infection is healed, it will stop the extra production of white blood cells.

Damaged Cells

DNA is a substance that helps to direct the activities of a cell. Every cell in our body has DNA. Should this DNA become damaged, a cell will either repair the DNA or it will die. Most often damaged DNA is caused by exposure to something in the environment, such as tobacco smoke. On rare occasions, damaged DNA can be inherited. Sometimes, cells with damaged DNA keep dividing even when new cells are not needed. These extra cells can form a mass that is sometimes called a growth or a **tumor**.

Cell

The smallest unit of living structure capable of independent existence. Cells are highly specialized in structure and function.

DNA (deoxyribonucleic acid)

A type of nucleic acid found principally in the nuclei of animal and plant cells; considered to be the autoreproducing component of chromosomes and many viruses as well as the repository for hereditary characteristics.

Tumor

Any swelling caused by an increased number of abnormal cells.

Tumors

Tumors can be benign or malignant. A **benign tumor** will stop growing and does not invade other tissues. An example of a benign tumor is a lipoma, which is a soft, fatty tumor that forms under the skin. Tumors classified as **malignant** are composed of cells different from normal cells in several important ways. Malignant, or cancerous, cells lose the ability to stop growing and dividing when they are no longer needed, which means that they keep multiplying. In addition, they also lose the ability to "mature" and do the job they were meant to do. These "immature" cells are often not useful to our body at all. For example, cancerous white blood cells are too immature to fight infection, but they continue to grow and divide even when they are not needed.

Cancerous cells can spread to other organs or parts of the body far from where the cancer originated. When cancerous cells leave their original location and invade other organs, the process is called **metastasis**. Cancerous cells can invade organs next to where they originated, or they can travel through the body's bloodstream or lymphatic system to reach distant locations. The location where the cancer started is called the **primary tumor**. For example, if a tumor starts in the lung but travels to the liver, it is said to be a primary lung cancer that has metastasized to the liver. Both locations have lung cancer cells and are treated by medications that are effective for lung cancer.

4. What is cancer of the esophagus?

Cancer of the esophagus is an abnormal growth of cells occurring within the esophagus. This growth can occur anywhere along the length of the esophagus. The most common location for cancer to develop is at the **gastroesophageal junction**, which is located at the bottom of the esophagus where it joins with the stomach.

THE BASICS

Benign tumor
A growth or mass of abnormal cells that does not invade or destroy adjacent normal tissue.

Malignant tumor
A rapid growth of abnormal cells that replaces normal cells, invades other tissues and organs, may recur after attempted removal, and is likely to cause the death of the host if left inadequately treated.

Metastasis
Transmission of cancer cells from an original site to one or more sites in the body.

Primary tumor
Location where the original tumor began.

Gastroesophageal junction
Location where the stomach and esophagus meet, also known as the cardia.

Squamous cell carcinoma

A malignant neoplasm derived from stratified squamous epithelium cells, such as those that line the esophagus.

Adenocarcinoma

A malignant neoplasm of epithelial cells in a glandular or gland-like pattern.

There are two main cell types of esophageal cancer: **squamous cell carcinoma** and **adenocarcinoma**. Squamous cell carcinoma arises in the cells that line the esophagus, and adenocarcinoma arises in the glandular cells of the esophagus. Squamous cell carcinomas usually occur in the upper and middle part of the esophagus, and adenocarcinomas usually occur in the lower part of the esophagus. Treatment options are the same for both types. The only way to be sure of the type of cancer is to have a biopsy reviewed by an experienced pathologist.

Other types of esophageal cancer are seen less frequently. On rare occasions, sarcoma, lymphoma, small cell carcinoma, mucoepidermoid carcinoma, adenoid cystic carcinoma, and spindle cell carcinoma are diagnosed in the esophagus. It also is possible that cancer starting in another part of the body can occasionally spread to the esophagus.

Bart's comment:

When I was told by my doctor in December of 1999 that I had cancer of the esophagus, it was a total shock. I remember saying to the doctor, "I wasn't aware that you could get cancer of the esophagus." Upon further contemplation of what the doctor had told me, I asked myself, "What information about this type of cancer could I have heeded, or what could I have done to possibly avoid this cancer?" And, in retrospect, there was nothing.

I realized that a person with chronic heartburn over a long period of time could be at risk for this cancer, and that was what I had over the last 15 years. Over-the-counter drugs did their job and the acid reflux would go away. I did not know this could possibly cause cancer, and I believe many people with chronic heartburn are unaware of this possibility. Part of my incentive to be part of this project and other efforts to distribute educational information is to let people recognize that this cancer exists, and they need to pay attention to this possibility.

5. How common is esophageal cancer?

Cancer of the esophagus is among the 10 most frequent cancers in the world, with more than 500,000 new cases each year. One type of esophageal cancer, squamous cell carcinoma, is prevalent in Asia (Turkey, Soviet Union, Iran, Iraq, and China), parts of Africa, and France. Adenocarcinoma of the esophagus has been rising dramatically in the United States and Western Europe, and is the type found in over 80% of patients diagnosed with esophageal cancer. A data analysis from the National Cancer Institute's SEER program found that from the early 1970s to the late 1980s the number of new cases of adenocarcinoma of the esophagus in white males has doubled. The causes for this alarming increase are unclear.

In the United States, approximately 15,500 new cases of esophageal cancer are diagnosed each year. Although cancer of the esophagus is fairly common in some parts of the world, in the United States it accounts for about 1% of all cancers.

6. What causes esophageal cancer?

The exact causes of cancer of the esophagus are not known, and researchers and doctors are actively working to identify them. The more they find out about what causes cancer of the esophagus, the better their chances will be of finding ways to prevent it. Avoiding tobacco entirely and drinking alcohol in moderation are lifestyle factors that may help to prevent the disease. Some factors that may place an individual at risk for the disease have been identified, but a direct cause is not yet known. (Information on risk factors for the disease is included in Part Two.)

Risk and Prevention

What are the risk factors for
esophageal cancer?

Is esophageal cancer hereditary?

What are the warning signs of
esophageal cancer?

Will taking heartburn medications help
prevent esophageal cancer?

More . . .

7. *What are risk factors?*

A risk factor is anything that increases an individual's chances of developing a disease. Some risk factors are external, such as the environment (exposure to chemicals) or lifestyle (smoking). We have some control over these external factors and may be able to change our health habits or environment to minimize our risk of disease. Other factors, like inherited genes or traits, are internal factors over which we have no control.

If you feel you may be at an increased risk for esophageal cancer, it is best to discuss this with your physician.

The presence of a risk factor does not mean that an individual will develop the disease. Also, some individuals develop a disease without having any of the suspected risk factors. In most cases, the disease may be the result of several factors, known and unknown. If you feel you may be at an increased risk for esophageal cancer, it is best to discuss this with your physician. He or she may be able to suggest ways to reduce the risk as well as assess your need for routine check-ups.

8. *What are the risk factors for esophageal cancer?*

Identifying the factors that place an individual at risk for esophageal cancer is the first step to preventing the disease. The risk factors for esophageal cancer are still being investigated, but some correlation has been found among the following factors.

Individual or Lifestyle Factors:

Age—The number of cases of esophageal cancer increases with age, with most cases found in individuals over age 55.

Gender—Cancer of the esophagus is three times more common in men than in women.

Race—Recently, a dramatic increase in new cases of adenocarcinoma of the esophagus has been seen in Caucasians. This prevalence is in contrast to squamous cell carcinoma, which is three times as common in African Americans as compared to Caucasians. The reason for this disparity is not clear.

Tobacco use—Individuals who smoke cigarettes or use smokeless tobacco tend to develop esophageal cancer more often than those who do not.

Alcohol use—Excessive use of alcohol can increase an individual's chance of developing this disease. Individuals who use both alcohol and tobacco have an increased risk of developing esophageal cancer. It is thought that each of these substances increases the harmful effects of the other.

Obesity—Individuals who are overweight or obese are more than two times as likely to develop adenocarcinoma than are individuals who are normal weight. The mechanism for the relationship between obesity and esophageal adenocarcinoma is not yet known, but increases in gastric reflux due to obesity may play a part in the increased risk.

Diet—Esophageal cancer may be associated with poor nutrition. Eating a diet low in fresh fruits and vegetables, and diets lacking in vitamins A, B_1, C, or beta-carotene, appears to contribute to the development of esophageal cancer. Researchers are not sure how diet increases the risk of developing esophageal cancer. It is important, however, to eat a well-balanced diet that includes fruits and vegetables. The American Cancer Society recommends eating five or more servings of vegetables and fruits each day, using whole grains such as brown rice and whole wheat instead of refined or processed grains, and limiting red meat.

Medical Conditions:

Reflux—Frequent and repeated reflux results in chronic heartburn, a condition called gastro-esophageal reflux disease (GERD; see Question 2). This chronic reflux can cause changes to the lower esophagus ranging from irritation of the lining (esophagitis) to ulceration, scarring, **stricture**, and Barrett's esophagus.

Barrett's esophagus—When cells lining the esophagus are irritated, they can change over time and begin to resemble the cells that line the stomach or the intestines, causing a condition known as Barrett's esophagus. The risk of developing Barrett's esophagus is 5 to 6 times higher for males than for females, and it is even greater for whites than for blacks. The incidence in Hispanics and Asians is very low. The possibility of cancer developing in the Barrett's esophagus is high and is estimated to be 1% to 2% per year (see Question 13).

Achalasia—In this condition, the muscles in the esophagus do not contract as they should. The sphincter at the lower end of the esophagus does not relax normally and the muscular activity in the esophagus is lost, resulting in retention of food in the esophagus. Esophageal cancer is more common in individuals with a history of achalasia.

Tylosis—In this rare inherited disease, excess skin grows on the palms of the hands and the soles of the feet. Individuals with this condition are at high risk to develop cancer of the esophagus and should be screened regularly.

Irritation of the esophagus—Swallowing substances that irritate the esophageal lining, such as lye or other caustic substances, can lead to significant damage and increase the risk of developing esophageal cancer years later.

Stricture

A narrowing or tightening of a hollow structure.

Medical history—Individuals who have had cancer of the head and neck have an increased chance of developing a second cancer, including esophageal cancer.

Research to identify additional risk factors and possible causes of esophageal cancer is ongoing. A number of factors are associated with higher incidence of esophageal cancer, but the exact cause and mechanism of development of esophageal cancer is not yet known. The risk factors we discussed may or may not lead to the development of esophageal cancer, and many people who have the disease do not have any risk factors. Lifestyle changes that can be made now to help prevent esophageal cancer include:

1. Quit smoking, do not start smoking, and do not use tobacco in any form.
2. Eat a balanced diet, including fruits, vegetables, and whole grains.
3. Drink alcohol in moderation.

Preliminary research has demonstrated that the risk of esophageal cancer may be lower in people who take aspirin or other non-steroidal anti-inflammatory drugs (NSAIDs), such as ibuprofen, but these associations need to be studied further.

Bart's comment:

A major risk factor in esophageal cancer is chronic heartburn (more than twice a week). If a person has had this condition for 6 months or longer, he should see his gastroenterologist. Smoking and drinking have been linked to esophageal cancer, as has obesity. People who smoke, drink excessively, have GERD, excessive heartburn, or indigestion, and do not maintain a balanced diet are at risk.

9. Is esophageal cancer hereditary?

The vast majority of individuals with esophageal cancer have no family history of esophageal cancer. At this time, there are no known genetic links to esophageal cancer, and there is no evidence that it can be passed on to the children of a person who has the disease. However, very rarely, there are families with more than one member who has developed esophageal cancer. Research is ongoing to identify possible causes and risk factors for this disease. If you are concerned about the disease, it is best to discuss these concerns with your family physician or a gastroenterologist.

Bart's comment:

Although there is no definite link from a hereditary point of view, some people who have contracted this disease have relatives within their families who have stomach and/or esophageal problems.

Until more information is known, it is best to have any symptoms evaluated by a physician.

10. What are the warning signs of esophageal cancer?

Early stage tumors rarely cause any symptoms and are therefore difficult to diagnose.

Unfortunately, diagnosis of esophageal cancer is usually made in advanced stages of disease when it becomes symptomatic. Diagnosis may be made at the time of an endoscopy for evaluation of symptoms such as heartburn, gastrointestinal bleeding, or surveillance of Barrett's esophagus. Early stage tumors rarely cause any symptoms and are therefore difficult to diagnose. The most common symptom is progressively worsening difficulty in swallowing, starting with solid foods and ultimately a complete blockage if untreated. The first symptom may be when food, often a piece of meat, gets "stuck" when trying to swallow. Difficulty in swallowing may present as a sensation of fullness, pressure, or burning. These problems may be intermittent or they may get progressively worse over time. Initial difficulty may be seen when eating meats, bread, or dry foods. In some patients, swallowing may also become painful. Loss of appetite due to the cancer itself or symptoms associated with diagnosis will often lead to weight loss. This weight loss often causes individuals to see their doctor prior to a diagnosis of esophageal cancer.

Patients may present with weakness, lack of energy, tiredness, or fatigue. Fatigue may be due to **anemia** caused by slow undetected bleeding from the tumor or to a compromised nutritional status.

As tumors block the esophagus, they may cause coughing due to **aspiration** of retained food and secretions in the esophagus. Aspiration also may occur due to paralysis of the vocal cords when the nerves to the vocal cords are involved by the tumor. In very advanced stages, tumors involving the upper esophagus may develop a communication or "**fistula**" (a tubular passageway) between the esophagus and the windpipe.

Cancer is just one potential cause of these symptoms. There can be a number of other, less serious medical conditions that may cause these symptoms. People with symptoms such as these should see their family doctor and a **gastroenterologist**. A gastroenterologist is a doctor who specializes in diseases of the digestive tract and is the appropriate medical professional to evaluate these symptoms.

Anemia

A condition in which the number of blood cells, amount of hemoglobin, and/or the volume of packed red blood cells is less than normal. Symptoms include pallor of the skin, shortness of breath, palpitations of the heart, and fatigue.

Aspiration

The inspiratory sucking into the airways of fluid or any foreign material, especially gastric contents.

Fistula

An abnormal passage from a hollow organ to the body surface or from one organ to another.

Gastroenterologist

A physician with special training in the function and disorders of the gastrointestinal system, including the stomach, intestines, and related organs of the gastrointestinal tract.

Bart's comment:

The problem with this disease is that the early signs can be masked by other non-crucial types of problems. Heartburn, which is considered a common problem that occurs in millions of Americans, can be an early sign of esophageal cancer. Persistent heartburn (over a 6- to 12-month period) should be discussed with your doctor and a gastroenterologist to see if this has gone beyond the simple problem to a more serious problem. Having difficulty swallowing or food occasionally getting stuck in your esophagus could be considered a late sign of this disease and should be evaluated by a physician immediately.

11. Are there any screening recommendations for esophageal cancer?

Currently there are no screening guidelines for the early detection of esophageal cancer. The challenge for doctors and researchers is to identify individuals who may be at higher risk to develop esophageal cancer. Research is ongoing to help determine which patients will benefit most from medical surveillance of esophageal disorders and symptoms.

It is important if you have any of the risk factors, such as chronic heartburn or reflux, that you see a physician or a gastroenterologist. These risk factors will probably not lead to esophageal cancer, but are uncomfortable to the individual experiencing them and may lead to other serious conditions. A gastroenterologist will be able to assess and manage your symptoms and can recommend the appropriate medical follow-up.

12. I have GERD. What should I do if the heartburn has lasted more than six months?

Heartburn is often described as a burning sensation behind the breastbone. It commonly occurs in the lower half of the esophagus but can occur all the way up to the throat. Many people will experience occasional heartburn or reflux, particularly after a spicy or high fat meal. Occasional heartburn is usually nothing to worry about, and there are many over-the-counter products to treat occasional heartburn. However, if symptoms persist for more than one month, you should see a doctor. Another common symptom is regurgitation, a backup of bitter-tasting fluid. These symptoms are usually worse after meals or when lying flat.

A diet high in fat or particular foods such as whole milk, citrus fruits, chocolate, mints, or tomatoes can lead to reflux. Eating large meals, smoking, alcohol consumption, or reclining after meals can also cause reflux. In addition, certain medical conditions such as a **hiatal hernia (Figure 2)**, pregnancy, and obesity can increase an individual's risk of developing reflux.

Heartburn that is persistent and lasts at least two days a week for more than six months could be a sign of a more serious condition known as gastroesophageal reflux disease or GERD, as discussed in Question 2. Approximately 20% of adults in the United States have symptoms of GERD. The esophagus is normally protected by a muscle located at the top of the stomach called the **lower esophageal sphincter (LES)**. This muscle keeps stomach acid from backing up into the esophagus. If this muscle is weakened, stomach contents are allowed to enter the esophagus. One reason why it may be weakened

Hiatal hernia

A condition in which part of the stomach protrudes through the esophageal opening (esophageal hiatus) of the diaphragm.

Lower esophageal sphincter (LES)

A muscle located at the top of the stomach that opens and closes to keep stomach acid and bile from backing up into the esophagus.

17

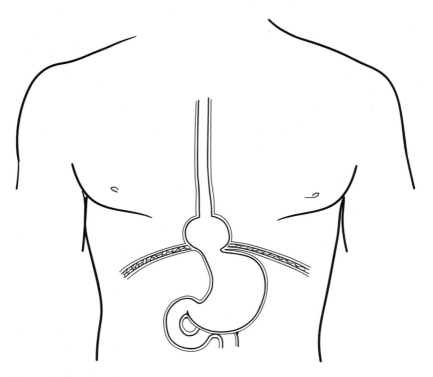

Figure 2 Hiatal hernia.

is a hiatal hernia. A hiatal hernia occurs when a small section of the upper part of the stomach slides back and forth between the chest and the abdomen. The stomach lining has a special protective barrier against acid, but the lining of the esophagus does not. If the lower esophageal sphincter does not function properly and acid enters the esophagus, it can cause an uncomfortable burning sensation (heartburn), which over time can lead to irritation, inflammation, and damage to the wall of the esophagus. Left untreated, GERD can cause complications such as esophagitis, which is an inflammation and erosion of the esophagus caused from exposure to stomach acid. A stricture, or scar tissue, can develop as a result of acid exposure and cause the esophagus to narrow. Barrett's esophagus is a condition where the lining of the esophagus actually changes in response to repeated acid exposure. Each of these conditions requires evaluation and follow-up with a physician.

You should see a physician if you have persistent heartburn. It may be best to see your family doctor, who can then refer you to a specialist (gastroenterologist) if necessary. Several symptoms are more urgent, however, and you should see a doctor immediately if you experience:

- Difficulty swallowing or feeling as if food is stuck in your throat
- Unexplained weight loss
- Chest pain
- Hoarseness
- Dark stools or blood in stools

Each of these symptoms may be a sign of a more serious condition and should be evaluated by a physician.

Bart's comment:
You should see a doctor if you have persistent reflux. A drug may be recommended that you should take for a stipulated period of time. If the problem continues once you stop taking the medicine, then you should see a gastroenterologist and possibly have an endoscopy done.

13. Tell me more about "Barrett's esophagus." What is it? What causes it?

Barrett's esophagus is a condition that occurs as a complication of chronic GERD. Over time, chronic reflux of the acidic stomach contents or bile into the esophagus leads to changes in the cells that line the esophagus. The acid changes the squamous cells that normally line the

You should see a physician if you have persistent heartburn.

esophagus so they are more like the lining of the stomach or the intestines. When viewed under a microscope, healthy tissue lining the esophagus is a whitish color. In an individual with Barrett's esophagus, the whitish lining has turned to an abnormal salmon-pink color. This change is called **metaplasia** and is most often seen near the gastroesophageal junction, where the esophagus meets the stomach. Metaplasia is the process of the replacement of one tissue lining by another type of tissue. This cellular change in the tissue is thought to be a protective response because the lining in Barrett's esophagus is more resistant to injury from acid than the original lining of the esophagus.

Barrett's esophagus does not have unique symptoms, and you will not even know you have it unless you have an **endoscopy**. The symptoms associated with GERD—heartburn and regurgitation—are often seen in an individual with Barrett's. However, not all individuals with Barrett's esophagus have symptoms of GERD.

Barrett's esophagus can only be diagnosed by an endoscopy and a **biopsy**. An endoscopy is a procedure performed by a gastroenterologist where a lighted scope is inserted through the mouth, and the lining of the esophagus is visualized. This lining is viewed by the gastroenterologist, who can biopsy the tissue at the same time. When the biopsy is viewed by an experienced **pathologist**, the presence of intestinal type cells (called goblet cells because of their shape) confirms the diagnosis of Barrett's esophagus. Both the visual change and the biopsy result are required for a diagnosis of Barrett's esophagus.

An endoscopic biopsy may be misleading if there is inflammation in the esophagus, and the biopsy erroneously may be reported to show **dysplasia** (see

Metaplasia

Transformation of an adult, fully-formed cell of one kind into an abnormal cell of another kind; an acquired condition.

Endoscopy

(also called esophagoscopy or EGD) Examination of the interior of a canal or hollow viscus by means of a special instrument called an endoscope; the patient is sedated during the process.

Biopsy

A process of removing tissue from a patient for diagnostic examination.

Pathologist

A physician who practices, evaluates, and/or supervises diagnostic tests, using materials removed from living or dead patients, to determine the causes or nature of the disease change.

Dysplasia

Abnormal development or growth of tissues, cells, or organs.

Question 18). If there is inflammation, it is important for you to be treated for reflux with high doses of proton pump inhibitors (such as Prilosec, Prevacid, or Nexium) and for the biopsy to be repeated. If there is no dysplasia in two consecutive biopsies, the American College of Gastroenterology's 1998 guidelines suggest an endoscopy and biopsy every two to three years.

About 10% of Americans who have GERD will go on to develop Barrett's esophagus. The risk to that 10% of developing esophageal cancer is about 0.5% a year. Individuals with Barrett's esophagus are at greater than average risk to develop esophageal cancer and should be followed closely by their doctors. The progression of Barrett's esophagus to cancer is a reasonably well-established phenomenon, with changes progressing from low-grade dysplasia to high-grade dysplasia and then to cancer. Reports indicate that of the patients with metaplasia who are on medication therapy, a proportion of them will be fine and the cells will not progress to cancer. This cell progression is not merely one way. In several studies, approximately 25% of patients who have low-grade dysplasia may have no dysplasia on subsequent exams. Similarly, some patients with high-grade dysplasia may regress into low-grade dysplasia or no dysplasia at all. Overall, in most cases there is progression toward cancer.

Pathologists can disagree about the definition of low-grade and high-grade dysplasia. It is important to have at least two pathologists review the slides and confirm the presence of a high-grade dysplasia before an invasive treatment is undertaken.

If a diagnosis of Barrett's esophagus is suspected but uncertain, it is best to obtain a second opinion at a center that has extensive experience with the disease. This can prevent you from worrying about your long-term risk of cancer or the need for additional medical tests if the diagnosis of Barrett's was incorrect. It can also allow you to start close surveillance for cancer if the diagnosis of Barrett's is confirmed. Barrett's esophagus is treated by treating the underlying cause: GERD.

14. Does having Barrett's esophagus or GERD increase my risk of developing cancer? What is H. pylori, and what part does it play in GI disorders?

Yes, Barrett's esophagus is associated with an increased risk of esophageal cancer. The type of cancer that occurs in individuals with Barrett's esophagus is called adenocarcinoma, which arises from the intestinal cells. Squamous cell carcinoma of the esophagus arises from the squamous cells that line a normal esophagus and is not associated with Barrett's esophagus.

Helicobacter pylori (H. pylori)

A specific type of curved or spiral microorganism (bacterium) that colonizes on the surface of mucus-secreting columnar cells, secretes urease (which causes infection), and along with other dietary factors, leads to gastritis and peptic ulcer disease of the stomach. It may play a role in the development of dysplasia and metaplasia of gastric mucosa and distal gastric adenocarcinoma.

Esophageal adenocarcinoma has been increasing in frequency for the past 20 years, primarily in white males. It is not known why this is occurring. One possibility is that there is a decrease in **Helicobacter pylori (H. pylori)** infections in the stomach. H. pylori is a type of bacteria that is the major cause of ulcers. It is a very common infection and causes no symptoms in most of the individuals who are affected by it. If the infection goes untreated, it can lead to progressive inflammation of the stomach. This inflammation leads to a decrease in acid secretion. Due to better public health measures, this infection is diminishing worldwide. Some researchers speculate that the decreased acid production as a result of the H. pylori infection may actually have a protective effect to the esophagus—so the decline of H. pylori infections, while helpful in reducing the incidence of ulcers, actually contributes (in theory) to the increase in cancers. However, this link has not been proven and is still under investigation.

It is thought that approximately 10% to 15% of individuals with chronic GERD will develop Barrett's esophagus. It is unknown why some people with chronic GERD develop the condition and others do not. It is also unknown why Caucasian males seem to be more at risk to develop Barrett's esophagus than any other group. Relatively few patients with Barrett's esophagus will develop adenocarcinoma of the esophagus. However, Barrett's esophagus does put an individual at higher risk for cancer, and routine surveillance is necessary. Periodic, routine endoscopy and biopsy are recommended procedures that can help to detect early cancers.

15. How are GERD and Barrett's esophagus treated?

The primary treatment for GERD and Barrett's is the suppression of acid reflux. Lifestyle changes may relieve some of the symptoms of GERD. The following list contains some suggestions that may help:

- Do not eat large meals; rather, eat small, frequent meals.
- Do not lie down for about two hours after eating.
- Avoid late night snacks.
- Avoid highly seasoned foods, acidic juices, alcohol abuse, peppermint, products with caffeine, and fatty foods.
- Avoid tobacco products in any form.
- To reduce reflux, sleep with the head of your bed raised 45 degrees.

- If you are overweight, losing weight will reduce reflux.
- If your doctor has prescribed medication for you, take it as directed.

Mild symptoms can be treated with over-the-counter medications such as antacids or low doses of medications called **H-2 blockers**. More persistent symptoms can be treated with higher doses of H-2 blockers. Examples of H-2 blockers are Tagamet, Pepcid, Zantac, and Axid. **Proton pump inhibitors** are medications used for ongoing therapy or complicated GERD (associated with bleeding or strictures). Examples of proton pump inhibitors are Prilosec, Prevacid, Aciphex, Protonix, and Nexium.

Proton pump inhibitors work by blocking the secretion of acid from the stomach. They can be effective in relieving heartburn and can allow the inflammation of the esophagus (esophagitis) to heal. Proton pump inhibitors are usually well tolerated and have minimal side effects. If you are taking any of these medications, it is important that you do not stop them suddenly. This can lead to an increase in symptoms. It is best to discuss your medications with a gastroenterologist who can change them if needed or instruct you on how to taper your dose.

16. Will taking heartburn medications help prevent esophageal cancer?

The long-term side effects of heartburn medications are still being investigated, and it is not known if they help to prevent esophageal cancer. Some laboratory studies have identified stomach tumors in rats after exposure to proton pump inhibitors; however, more than 15 years of experience with these medications has not identified a similar occurrence in humans. Some individuals on long-term medication therapy develop small benign

H-2 blocker

Type of pharmaceutical drug used to treat GERD and Barrett's esophagus; examples include Tagamet, Pepcid, Zantac, and Axid.

Proton pump inhibitor

Type of pharmaceutical drug used to treat more complicated GERD (associated with bleeding or strictures); examples include Prilosec, Prevacid, Aciphex, Protonix, and Nexium.

polyps in the stomach. These polyps do not become cancerous and cause no problems.

17. Is surgery used to treat GERD and Barrett's esophagus?

GERD, with or without Barrett's esophagus, is sometimes treated by surgery. This type of operation is called **fundoplication** or anti-reflux surgery, and is performed to stop the reflux of acid into the esophagus. The operation involves wrapping the stomach around the lower part of the esophagus, which tightens the lower esophageal sphincter and is intended to prevent reflux. These operations are typically performed by thoracic (chest) surgeons, gastric surgeons, or general surgeons. It is most often done laparoscopically, without the need for a large incision. **Laparoscopy** is a type of surgery where the surgeon inserts several tiny telescopes thru the abdomen. The abdomen is then inflated with carbon dioxide to move the abdominal wall away from the internal organs. The surgeon can then work with instruments, visualizing the area through the telescopes to perform the surgery.

Your doctor will need to do several tests to determine if you are a candidate for this type of surgery. Most patients who have the surgery have serious complications from GERD and require high doses of medications. There is no evidence that this type of surgery reduces the risk of esophageal cancer.

18. I've been told that I have high-grade dysplasia. What does this mean?

Dysplasia is the development of changes within a cell that are not normally seen in cells in that part of the body. Cells that have these dysplastic changes appear

Polyp

A general term used for any mass of tissue that bulges or projects outward or upward from the normal surface level; it is visible as a roundish structure growing from a mound-like base or a slender stalk.

Fundoplication

Suture of the fundus of the stomach completely or partly around the gastroesophageal junction to treat gastroesophageal reflux disease.

Laparoscopy

A type of surgery using a laparoscope, comprised of fiber optics and low-heat halogen bulbs that aid in the placement and use of other surgical tools. One or more tiny incisions enable precise incision, drainage, excision, cautery, ligation, suturing, and other surgical procedures.

RISK AND PREVENTION

malignant but do not invade other tissues like cancer cells. It is not yet known which patients with Barrett's esophagus will progress to dysplasia and which patients with dysplasia will progress to cancer.

Dysplasia is considered premalignant and is classified as high-grade, low-grade, or indefinite. The indefinite classification means that the pathologist is unable to tell if low-grade dysplasia is present or not. For low-grade and indefinite dysplasias, routine endoscopic biopsy surveillance is recommended. On the follow-up endoscopy, some patients will be found not to have dysplasia or will be diagnosed as having lesser grades of dysplasia. This change may represent a sampling variation or actual biological reversal. The exact reasons why the dysplasia may regress are not currently known.

The presence of high-grade dysplasia indicates that cancer may already be present, and surgery is the recommended treatment. Some patients with high-grade dysplasia may opt for follow-up biopsy surveillance. This is an important decision you should make only after a thorough discussion of the risks and benefits with a gastroenterologist and a thoracic surgeon. If you choose surveillance, it will be recommended that you have an endoscopy every three months for a year and then every four to six months afterward. The reason surgery is recommended instead of close follow-up is that there is high likelihood that cancer may be missed by the biopsies.

If you are diagnosed with high-grade dysplasia, your gastroenterologist may repeat your endoscopy with more biopsies. If you are diagnosed with Barrett's esophagus with dysplasia, it is important that a pathologist experienced in this diagnosis review your pathology slides. It is a common practice to ask a second or a third pathologist to review the pathology slides. This is important to check for agreement among pathologists and to possibly get a more experienced opinion. The presence of a risk factor does not mean that an individual will develop the disease.

PART THREE

Diagnosis and Staging

How is esophageal cancer diagnosed?

What tests are performed to aid in the diagnosis?

What does my doctor mean by "stage of disease," and why is staging important?

More . . .

19. How is esophageal cancer diagnosed?

Most patients with esophageal cancer are diagnosed after they experience symptoms and go to their doctor to be evaluated. They may go to their primary physician complaining that food is getting "stuck" during swallowing. Depending on the physician, she or he will either evaluate these symptoms personally or refer the patient to a specialist such as a gastroenterologist for evaluation. Either way, if an abnormality is identified, an endoscopy and biopsy are performed.

It is not unusual for an early stage cancer to be discovered during a routine endoscopy.

It is not unusual for an early stage cancer to be discovered during a routine endoscopy. People who suffer from heartburn or GERD or have been diagnosed with Barrett's esophagus often have an endoscopy periodically to monitor potential damage to the esophagus.

Bart's comment:

When I complained to my doctor that a piece of meat had gotten stuck in my esophagus and there was significant pain, we did an endoscopy, and that determined that I had a tumor in my esophagus. We did a CAT scan and a PET scan to confirm the cancer and to see if there were any other cancer sites in my body. Once we determined that this was the only cancer site, we then began the plan on how we would attack this cancer. A discussion with the team of doctors produced a chemotherapy and radiation protocol, followed by a surgery plan.

20. What tests are performed to aid in the diagnosis?

A number of tests are used to diagnose esophageal cancer. In most cases, multiple tests are required to fully evaluate the extent of the cancer. Each test will give the physicians different information.

- A **barium swallow** (also called an upper GI series or esophagram) is a type of radiology exam where you are asked to drink a barium solution before an x-ray is taken. This is often the first test done when a doctor is concerned about a problem in the esophagus. The barium coats the esophagus and stomach and shows up on an x-ray. The x-ray pictures will show the **radiologist** changes in the shape of the esophagus, stomach, and duodenum (the lower part of the stomach). It is often ordered to determine if and where in the esophagus an abnormality is located and if there is obstruction of the esophagus.

  A barium swallow is also used to identify such conditions as ulcers, hernias, blockages, and other abnormalities.

  In order to obtain a clear picture of your gastrointestinal system, you will be asked to not eat or drink anything for four to eight hours prior to the test. You will also be asked to remove any metallic objects, such as jewelry.

  Barium can cause constipation as it moves through the digestive system. To help minimize this, drink extra fluids after the test and ask your doctor if you should take a laxative. Barium has a whitish color and may be noticeable in your stools for several days after the test.

- A **CAT (computerized axial tomography) scan** of the chest and abdomen is often performed to assess for any anatomical abnormalities. A CAT scan is an x-ray procedure that uses a computer to generate cross-sectional views of the body. The pictures generated from a CAT scan show a "slice" of the body. An example often used to illustrate the type of images

Barium swallow

(also called upper GI series or esophagram) A type of radiology examination where a barium solution is drunk before the x-ray is taken to be able to visualize the esophagus, stomach, and duodenum.

Radiologist

A physician specially trained in the diagnostic and/or therapeutic use of x-rays and radionuclides, radiation physics, and biology; also trained in diagnostic ultrasound and magnetic resonance imaging and applicable physics.

Computerized axial tomography (CAT) scan

A type of x-ray procedure that is painless and provides multiple pictures of the body in specific sections for diagnostic purposes.

of a CAT scan is that of a loaf of bread. Imagine the body as a loaf of bread and you are looking at one end of the loaf. As each slice of bread is removed, you can see the entire surface of the next slice. Similarly, CAT scan images give physicians multiple pictures of your body, which help to define normal and abnormal structures. CAT scans are painless and may be done with intravenous (IV) and/or oral contrast, which will help to enhance the pictures. Your physician will look for thickening of the wall of the esophagus or stomach; any enlarged lymph nodes, lung, or liver nodules; and fluid in the chest or abdomen. The CAT scan is usually done on both the chest and the abdomen.

- An endoscopy (also called esophagoscopy or EGD) is a test done under sedation. It is performed to visualize the esophagus and to obtain biopsies. The physician (usually a gastroenterologist) will take a small flexible, lighted tube and insert it through your mouth to your esophagus. The physician can then visualize the inside of the esophagus and take a biopsy of any suspicious area. An endoscopy is sometimes done with ultrasound or sound waves (**endoscopic ultrasound or EUS**) to see how far into the wall of the esophagus the tumor has grown and to determine if any lymph nodes are involved.

Endoscopic ultrasound or EUS

A type of endoscopy that uses sound waves for diagnostic purposes.

An endoscopy and endoscopic ultrasound are valuable procedures in the diagnosis and staging of esophageal cancer. The ultrasound is actually able to see through the wall of the esophagus with much more accuracy than a CAT scan. The depth of the tumor into the wall of the esophagus is an important factor in considering the appropriate treatment for you. An endoscopic ultrasound is the best method to determine this depth. An endoscopic ultrasound can also see any enlarged lymph nodes or suspicious lymph nodes present along the esophagus or in the stomach. It is a relatively new technique, and not all gastroenterologists who perform endoscopy may perform endoscopic ultrasounds.

The gastroenterologist will be able to discuss the visual findings from the exam that day. If any biopsies were taken, these may require several days to be read by a pathologist. Your doctor will let you know when to expect any biopsy results.

- An endobronchial ultrasound or EBUS is a new diagnostic tool that combines two procedures (bronchoscopy and ultrasonography) to allow physicians to obtain precise biopsies of lymph nodes in the chest. It is an outpatient procedure and may be used to assess lymph nodes in the chest.

- A **Positron Emission Tomography (PET) scan** is used to determine the metabolic activity of different tissues and whether or not an abnormality is likely to be a cancer. Cancer cells are usually more active than normal cells and are presumed to metabolize nutrients faster. This difference in metabolism can be identified by a PET scan. A PET scan assesses the entire body for evidence of cancer and utilizes an injection that works with the glucose in the body to identify areas that are likely to be a cancer. An abnormal focus of increased activity may suggest the possibility of cancer at that site. A PET scan is a relatively new test but has quickly become a valuable tool to help physicians identify areas that may be of concern.

To prepare for this test, you will be asked to refrain from eating and drinking anything (except water) and to refrain from vigorous physical activity for several hours before the test. The reason for this is that the injection that is utilized for a PET scan works with the glucose in your body. Eating sugar (even a

PET (positron emission tomography) scan

A type of scan that measures positron-emitting isotopes with short half-lives that the patient has ingested to assess metabolic and physiologic function rather than anatomic structure.

piece of gum or candy) may interfere with the results of the test. After you receive the injection, you will be asked to lie in a quiet room for about 45 minutes. After this time, you will be placed on a moveable table where the scan will take place. Your doctor should receive the results of the test in several days. PET scans complement the other staging tests you are having. In about 15% to 20% of patients, a PET scan detects cancer that has spread beyond the esophagus. In addition, some recent research suggests that the level of activity measured by PET scan (often reported as Standard Uptake Value or SUV) is suggestive of prognosis.

Each of these tests will help your doctor to assess your condition. Each can identify an abnormality, but only with a biopsy can your physician say for sure whether it is a cancer or not. As your doctor orders tests, it is a good idea to check with your insurance company to determine whether you need pre-certification or authorization prior to having the test.

Bart's comment:

I was surprised at all of the tests they had available to further define this cancer and to see if there were any other tumors in my body. My suggestion would be that if you have had an initial diagnosis, you should go through a CAT scan, PET scan, and endoscopy before a plan is decided on by your medical team.

21. What does my doctor mean by "stage of disease," and why is staging important?

Your doctor will determine the stage of your disease for several important reasons. By "stage," he or she is referring to the extent of the cancer in your body. This includes where it is located, how extensive it is, and whether it has spread to any lymph nodes, nearby organs, or elsewhere in your body. Treatment for esophageal cancer includes **chemotherapy**, radiation therapy, surgery, or a combination of any or all of these. The stage of the disease will determine what treatment option will be the most suitable for you. Staging also gives physicians a standard language to discuss your treatment with other medical professionals involved in your care.

Chemotherapy
The use of drugs to kill cancer cells.

Bart's comment:

When we had all of the tests done, the doctors told me that I had a stage 3 tumor with no lymph node involvement.

22. How is esophageal cancer staged?

All solid tumors use a classification called the TNM staging system. *T* relates to the primary tumor, *N* indicates whether the lymph nodes are involved, and *M* denotes the presence or absence of metastasis. Once each of these areas has been evaluated by tests such as a CAT scan, endoscopic ultrasound, or PET scan, an overall stage is assigned. The overall stages are provided in the list that follows (see also **Figure 3**).

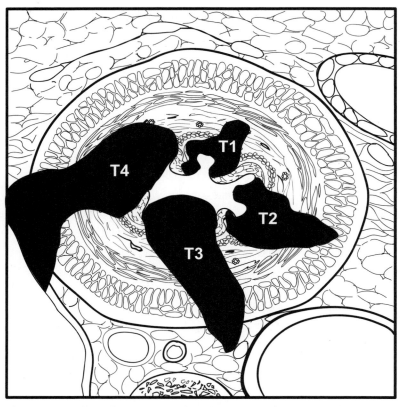

Figure 3 Esophageal cancer staging. Darkened areas demonstrate the level of invasion through the esophageal wall for each tumor stage.

- Stage I—the tumor is localized to the top few layers of the esophageal wall.
- Stage II—the tumor has invaded deeper into the esophageal wall and may involve local lymph nodes.
- Stage III—the tumor has invaded the full thickness of the wall of the esophagus or involves local lymph nodes.
- Stage IV—the tumor has spread beyond the esophagus to involve other parts of the body.

23. What are lymph nodes?

Lymph is an almost clear fluid that drains waste from cells. This fluid travels through vessels to our lymph nodes, which are small, bean-shaped structures located throughout our bodies that filter unwanted substances, such as cancer cells and bacteria, from the fluid. Since the job of the lymph nodes is to filter unwanted substances, like cancer cells, it is important to check them at diagnosis and during treatment (see **Figure 4**).

24. Why are lymph nodes important in esophageal cancer?

Whether the cancer has spread to the lymph nodes is an important factor to consider when deciding the best treatment for you. Lymph nodes may appear enlarged on diagnostic tests such as a CAT scan or an endoscopic ultrasound. A biopsy is required to know if they are involved with cancer or if they are enlarged for another reason, such as an infection. At the time of surgery, your surgeon may remove your lymph nodes as part of the operation. This is done for surgical staging, and some surgeons believe that the removal of lymph nodes near the area of the tumor improves survival following surgery.

25. How important are survival statistics to an individual patient?

Survival statistics for esophageal cancer are not very encouraging and can be overwhelming when viewed from an individual perspective. It is therefore imperative that one understands how these statistics are compiled.

Survival statistics for esophageal cancer can be overwhelming when viewed from an individual perspective.

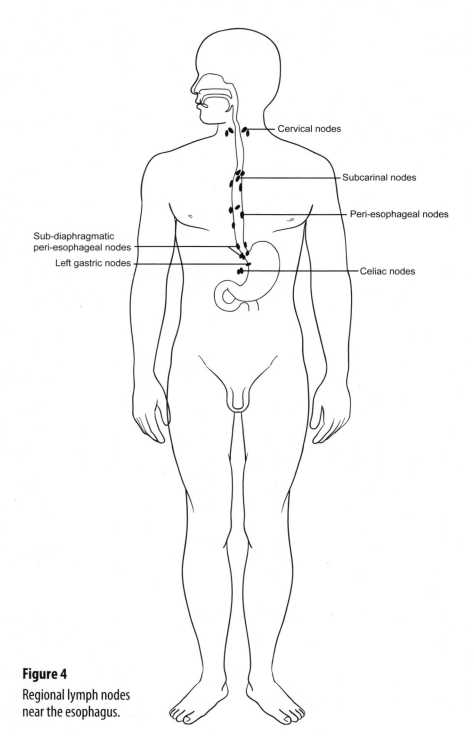

Figure 4

Regional lymph nodes near the esophagus.

Survival statistics measure the five-year survival rate of all patients with a similar diagnosis, but they cannot predict prognosis in a single individual. Your survival depends on a number of factors, including the stage of your disease, how well you respond to treatment, and your overall medical health. You should also keep in mind that the statistics you are viewing were compiled on therapies and technology that are often outdated. Treatment for esophageal cancer has changed dramatically over the past decades, and published statistics may not reflect improved treatment advances.

Bart's comment:

When you are dealing with cancer statistics as to life expectancy given your respective cancer, there is always a concern, and the number is of interest to the patient. When the doctor tells you that statistics indicate that there is a 20% chance you will live 5 years or that 3 out of 4 people who contract this cancer die from it, these are shocking comments. But do they really apply to me as a patient hearing them?

One must look at the individuals who are part of the database that gave rise to these statistics. What are the ages of those in the statistical database? Are they all 61 like myself, or are some older and some younger? If a database states "white males between 55 and 75," then this immediately raises questions as to the validity of that database because I am 61, and how do people at other ages affect these statistics? Mine was a stage 3 cancer. What were the stages of the other patients in this statistical base and how do they fare? Do they add to the life expectancy or take from it? The comparisons can go on and on. Were the participants in this statistical base smokers or drinkers, or were they sickly all their lives, or did they have stressful jobs versus people who have no stress in their lives? What I am trying to say is that most statistical databases do not specifically apply exactly to you, and therefore, as I like to say, "YOU ARE A STATISTIC OF ONE!"

All the statistics in the world do not compensate for the will of the individual to meet this challenge and actively fight this problem and beat the odds. "Problems are opportunities," a boss once told me, and having been told you have cancer is all you need to know to say, "I am going to meet this challenge and I will win. I will never give up."

Having a positive attitude goes a long way in fighting this disease. For you to stay in control, make sure you are a part of the decision process, and make sure you retain that positive attitude through all the treatments you have to endure. I am sure you will have positive outcome. God made each of us unique, and no two of us are exactly the same; it is this uniqueness that makes us special.

PART FOUR

Coping with the Diagnosis

I've been diagnosed with esophageal cancer.
What should I do now?

How do I select a surgeon or medical oncologist?

Should I get a second opinion?

More . . .

26. I've been diagnosed with esophageal cancer. What should I do now?

If you've been diagnosed with cancer of the esophagus, you already may have been seeing your family doctor or a gastroenterologist. These physicians should explain to you what they think the next best step will be. An evaluation by a physician who specializes in esophageal cancer will be important in planning your care. Esophageal cancer is a rare type of cancer, and it may be necessary to go to a larger university hospital to see doctors who have experience treating esophageal cancer. It will be beneficial to see both a medical **oncologist** (a doctor who treats cancer with medications such as chemotherapy) and a surgical oncologist. Esophageal cancer is often treated in a **multimodal** fashion, and each of these specialists can offer their opinion as to the best treatment course for you. Radiation is often used to treat esophageal cancer, and a medical oncologist or surgical oncologist can refer you to a radiation oncologist for treatment if necessary.

When making plans to see a specialist, it is helpful to collect a copy of any physician's notes, test results, radiology reports and films, and any other medical information related to your diagnosis and past medical history. It is very important for the doctors to see the actual radiology films in addition to the paper report. The doctors you will be seeing will need a copy of your records, and it may save time and energy to ask for a copy of each report as you have each test rather than gathering all the information at a later date. If you have had a biopsy at a different hospital from the one at which you will be treated, you will probably be required to bring in the glass slides made from your original biopsy. Most hospitals require review of previous biopsies by their pathologists prior to starting treatment or having surgery. The patient is

Oncologist

A physician with specialized training in the science of the physical, chemical, and biological properties of neoplasms, including causation, pathogenesis, and treatment.

Multimodality

The use of specialists in two or more disciplines to treat a specific disease; may include diagnostic testing, radiation, pharmaceuticals, or surgery.

responsible for obtaining the slides and pathology report from the hospital that performed the biopsy. If your primary care physician has been coordinating your care, his or her office may be able to help obtain some of this information.

Bart's comment:

The first step in the process is to determine the institution that has experience treating this kind of cancer. Visiting Web sites of the different cancer centers will give you insight into the facility the particular center has, the attention they pay to thoracic cancers, and the team they have assembled to handle this kind of cancer.

27. How do I select a surgeon or medical oncologist?

It is important to be sure that you are getting the best care possible, and this starts with your choice of doctors. A recommendation from a reliable source, such as your primary care physician or gastroenterologist, is a good place to start. You can also call the nearest cancer center or university hospital to find a specialist. The National Cancer Institute (NCI) has a toll free phone number (1-800-4-CANCER) that you can call to find a specialist near you. The leading cancer centers are identified by the National Cancer Institute as NCI-designated comprehensive cancer centers. The American College of Surgeons' Web site (*http://www.facs.org*) lists its members by specialty. At the main page of their Web site, you can go to the "public and press" tab, and from there you can search for members with a specialty in thoracic surgery or general surgery, or for a surgeon located near you. The American Society of Clinical Oncology also has a Web site, CancerNet (*http://www.cancer.net*). From the main

It is important to be sure that you are getting the best care possible, and this starts with your choice of doctors.

page, you can go to "For patients, families, and friends" and then use the quick links to search for a medical oncologist, radiation oncologist, or surgeon near you.

After you have identified a specific doctor, it is important to evaluate whether this person is a qualified physician and whether you are comfortable with him or her. Some things to consider include:

- Clinical experience—It will be critical to determine whether a physician has experience with the treatment of esophageal cancer. Oncologists treat patients with all types of cancer, but ideally you want to find one who specializes in esophageal cancer. Surgical oncologists also may treat many types of cancer, so it is helpful to look for one who has experience with esophageal cancer. You should also ask the physicians what percentage of their practice is esophageal cancer and how many esophageal surgeries they perform over a given amount of time (i.e., within a year).
- Hospital affiliation—Cancer centers and university hospitals conduct research and provide access to the newest treatments and clinical trials. They also have experience with less common types of cancer such as esophageal cancer. When choosing a physician, keep in mind that you are not only choosing the physician, but also the nursing and ancillary staff. You should feel comfortable and confident with the entire team who will be helping to take care of you.
- Credentials—Basic professional information for licensed U.S. physicians is available through the American Medical Association's Doctor Finder Web site (*http://webapps.ama-assn.org/doctorfinder/html/patient.html*). At the Web site, you can search by physician's name or specialty. Each listing offers information on the physician's medical school, residency and

fellowship training, board certification, and office location. Board certification ensures proficiency in a specified area, such as medical oncology, radiation oncology, general surgery, or thoracic surgery. Residency or fellowship training at a major cancer center can be a plus, as that involves rigorous post-graduate education with experts in the field of oncology.

Other factors that you should also consider:

- Finances—Is the doctor covered by your insurance plan? Financial constraints are a reality, and insurance coverage should be considered when selecting a doctor. Your doctors should be covered under your policy unless cost is not an issue for you. However, there may be reasons you need to see a specialist outside your insurance plan. Esophageal cancer is a relatively rare form of cancer and not every doctor or surgeon has experience treating it. In some cases, insurance companies may make exceptions for coverage to a specialist not participating in your policy. It may be helpful to speak with a **social worker** at the hospital where you are being treated or the benefits representative at your place of employment if you cannot find a specialist in your plan who treats esophageal cancer or if you have questions regarding insurance issues. You may also want to call your insurance company to see about out-of-network coverage.

- Distance—Treatment for esophageal cancer, such as chemotherapy or radiation therapy, may require multiple, or even daily, trips to the doctor or hospital. Surgery usually requires an extended hospital stay. If you feel this may become a significant issue for you and your family, it may be helpful to speak with the hospital's social worker about transportation alternatives or possibilities for inexpensive lodging.

Social worker

A degreed mental health professional who can provide counseling services to individuals and groups as well as help the patient network with community services and resources.

Bart's comment:

Once you have selected the cancer center, you need to evaluate the surgeons and medical oncologists associated with that cancer center. Reputation and years of service play a role in your selection. Also, frequency at which the surgery is performed at this center is important to know and, more specifically, how many surgeries of this nature the surgeon you are thinking about has performed.

28. Who are the other members of the medical team? What is multidisciplinary care?

Esophageal cancer is a complex disease, and its treatment frequently involves some combination of surgery, chemotherapy, and radiation. You likely will see more than one specialist for your esophageal cancer care, including medical oncologists, thoracic surgeons, radiation oncologists, and dietitians. Ideally, these specialists work together in a multidisciplinary setting where they can easily consult with each other and reach a consensus about your treatment options. This multidisciplinary approach not only offers you high-quality care, but also has practical advantages that may include fewer trips to the doctor, less time from diagnosis to start of treatment, and more efficient coordination of treatment logistics. Multidisciplinary care is commonly offered in cancer centers and in larger treatment centers such as university hospitals, but it is beginning to be implemented in some community hospitals as well.

Each specialist you see is a member of your treatment team, but one doctor will have primary responsibility for managing and directing your care. There are also a number of other doctors, along with support staff, who will be involved in your care. It is helpful to understand what each of these healthcare professionals does, and what role he or she plays in your care. The following list contains a brief description of healthcare professionals who may be involved in your care.

- Medical oncologist: a physician who performs comprehensive management of cancer patients throughout all phases of care. Medical oncologists specialize in treating cancer with medicine, using systemic treatments such as chemotherapy.

- Surgical oncologist: a physician who specializes in performing cancer surgery. Some surgeons have received additional training in chest surgery and are considered thoracic surgeons.

- Radiation oncologist: a physician who specializes in treating cancer with radiation.

- Gastroenterologist: a physician who specializes in diagnosis and treatment of gastrointestinal diseases.

- Pathologist: a physician trained to examine and evaluate cells and tissue. The pathologist evaluates your biopsy tissue and furnishes a biopsy report to your oncologist or surgeon.

- Oncology nurse: a specialized nurse trained to provide care to cancer patients, including administering chemotherapy and monitoring side effects.

- Psychiatrist: a physician who specializes in treating people for depression, anxiety, and other psychological illness. Psychiatrists provide psychotherapy and can also prescribe medication.

- Psychologist: a person trained in psychology who can provide psychotherapy.

- Oncology social worker: a social worker trained to provide counseling and practical assistance to cancer patients. Social workers can help you locate services such as transportation, support groups, and home care. They can also provide assistance with insurance and financial issues.

- Rehabilitation specialist: a person trained to help patients recover from physical changes brought about by cancer or cancer treatment. Physical therapists can help patients recover range of motion and strength following esophageal surgery.

Dietitian

A degreed professional who can develop a nutritious eating plan for an individual.

- Nutritionist or **dietitian**: a person trained to provide nutritional or dietary counseling. Patients with esophageal cancer may experience weight loss as a result of their cancer or its treatment. Treatment side effects, such as nausea from chemotherapy or heartburn from radiation, can negatively affect appetite. Nutritional or dietary counseling services can help patients to increase appetite and gain weight.

Bart's comment:

My team at MSKCC was comprised of Dr. Bains my surgeon, Dr. Ilson my medical oncologist, and Dr. Minsky my radiologist. I referred to them as the IBM of Memorial-Sloan Kettering Cancer Center.

29. Should I get a second opinion?

A second opinion is a good way to be sure you are receiving the best possible care while having peace of mind that you have explored all of your options.

The quality of the care you will receive is very important. A second opinion is a good way to be sure you are receiving the best possible care while having peace of mind that you have explored all of your options. A second opinion can offer new options, confirm recommendations, or bring to light substandard care. It is a good idea to check with your insurance company prior to getting a second opinion. They may be able to help you find a specialist who is covered by your plan.

A second opinion requires some logistics—everything you gathered for your first appointment will also be needed for a second opinion.

There are certain instances when a second opinion is particularly important:

- If you have been told you are not a candidate for surgery but you have reason to think you may be. Surgery offers the best chance for a cure, and decisions regarding who is an appropriate surgical candidate are changing and may differ from surgeon to surgeon.

- If a doctor tells you there are no treatment options. This is rarely the case, and a second opinion may bring additional choices for treatment. Larger hospitals or cancer centers may have access to new treatments through clinical trials that may benefit you.

- You should have a second opinion if you are uncomfortable with your doctor or have doubts about his or her recommendations for your care. It is vital to have a good doctor–patient relationship, and you should look for a doctor in whom you have confidence and with whom you are comfortable.

If you do get a second opinion and receive conflicting advice, seeking a third opinion or the advice of another doctor (such as your primary care doctor) can help to resolve any outstanding issues.

It is important to keep in mind that getting a second opinion can be emotionally draining and may consume time and energy you do not have. It may even create confusion and delay treatment. It is important to consider this prior to getting another opinion. A second opinion may or may not be covered by your insurance company and you may incur additional costs.

Some patients worry that they will offend a doctor by getting a second opinion. It is your right to seek a second opinion. If you sense that your doctor is threatened by your intention to get a second opinion, you might consider that to be reason enough to pursue another perspective.

Bart's comment:

Any major procedure or life-changing illness should be verified with a second opinion. However, time is of the essence, and it may take an unreasonable time to get a valid second opinion. At this point you need to determine how confident you are in the first opinion, if you feel comfortable with the hospital's experience and the surgeon's credentials, and how your meeting with the surgeon left you. If there is uncertainty, then wait for a second opinion. If you are comfortable with what you have heard and found out, then it would be prudent to proceed.

30. What questions should I ask my doctor?

This book will provide you with information that may prompt questions you would like to ask your doctor. It is always helpful to write down any questions you think of before you see the doctor to ensure that all of your questions are addressed. Listen to what the doctor has to say, since he or she may answer many of your questions when talking, and then ask any additional questions that were not covered. Having a close friend or family member with you during the visit is also very helpful. The more minds that are listening and asking questions, the better the chance your concerns will be addressed. It may also help to take notes during the conversation. Be sure you understand what the extent of your disease is (stage) and what treatment your doctor is recommending and why.

Bart's comment:

You should ask him how many of these operations he has done in the last six months and, perhaps more importantly, how many the hospital has done in that same period. After surgery, the hospital staff will be taking care of you, and knowing you are in the hands of a capable staff can rest your mind and speed your recovery.

31. How can I relate best to my doctor? What can I do to make my medical visits as productive as possible?

The doctor–patient relationship lies at the heart of patient care. This relationship will guide and support you throughout the course of your esophageal cancer. It is your job, and your doctor's, to nurture this relationship and to work toward a partnership based on mutual trust and respect. Although difficulties between doctor and patient may occur at times, just as they do in any relationship, these problems will be minimized if good communication is maintained. Remember that your doctor is not a mind reader. It is your responsibility to be open and honest in your communications and to bring up any concerns, needs, or preferences you may have. It is especially important that you feel comfortable discussing sensitive issues such as your use of alternative medicine treatments, your lifestyle (smoking, drinking, drugs), end-of-life issues, and sexual concerns. Keep in mind that conversations between doctor and patient are confidential and that the more your doctor knows about issues that may impact your health, the better care you will receive.

Although difficulties between doctor and patient may occur at times, just as they do in any relationship, these problems will be minimized if good communication is maintained.

At your first visit, you should address the issues of how much information you want from your doctor and how involved you would like to be in the decisions that are made about your care. Some patients want to know every-thing about their condition, and they want to make all of the decisions themselves. Some patients find too much information anxiety-provoking. These patients would prefer to hear less information (often only the good news) and are more comfortable allowing their doctor to make all the decisions. Many patients fall somewhere in between. Whatever your preferences may be, and they may change over time, it is your responsibility to com-municate them to your doctor. If you feel that your doctor is not responsive to your needs, or if you have other con-cerns regarding your relationship, you should bring them up before they reach a crisis stage. If you and your doctor cannot resolve disagreements in a productive and satis-factory manner, you should look for another doctor.

Think about what you are going to say to your doctor ahead of time. Remember, he or she has a finite amount of time to spend with you, so before your appointment consider which concerns are most pressing and write them down in order of importance. This tactic will help you focus and make the most effective use of the limited time you have with your doctor. If you choose to review events in great detail, you risk running out of the time that your doctor has for addressing your critical questions.

If you have symptoms to report, describe them clearly and concisely. Be prepared to answer your doctor's ques-tions, such as when the symptoms started, how often they occur, and how long they last. Don't be afraid to mention the emotional and social issues that are affecting you, in addition to any physical problems you have.

Always bring someone with you to your appointment. It is impossible to remember all that is said during an office visit, and emotions can cloud what a patient hears. It helps to have someone else along who can write down what the doctor says. It is important to understand everything your doctor tells you. If something is unclear, say so, and ask questions until you are satisfied that you understand completely.

Be sure that all necessary tests are completed prior to your visit and that you have all the information you need. This includes having the required referrals, if any, and a current list of the prescriptions and nonprescription drugs you are taking. Bring a notebook or binder to each appointment that contains your medical information and paperwork. If you can present your doctor with the information needed to care for you in an efficient and clear manner, you will go a long way toward increasing the quality of your relationship with your doctor and, ultimately, the quality of your care.

Bart's comment:

In my case I wanted to remain in control and wanted to make all the decisions. We would discuss what they wanted to do and why and left it to me to make that final decision. Staying in control and working with your team in my mind is essential. An informed patient and caregiver will lead to a better relationship with the medical team you have selected.

32. Can exercise help me cope with diagnosis and treatment?

Studies have shown that engaging in some form of moderate exercise helps one both physically and mentally. Simply walking for twenty to thirty minutes daily can increase appetite, lift your spirits, and increase energy.

All forms of treatment are a drain on energy stores, both physically and emotionally, and it is important to stay as fit as possible.

Exercise becomes even more important when undergoing cancer therapy. All forms of treatment are a drain on energy stores, both physically and emotionally, and it is important to stay as fit as possible. Fatigue is a common symptom during and after cancer treatment, and physical activity can help to reduce this fatigue. Starting with a slow exercise program, such as walking, can help to restore energy. There will be days, however, when you will be just too fatigued for any form of exercise. Do not push your body further than it can go, but remember to resume your exercise routine when you are able. If your fatigue persists, see your doctor. Sometimes fatigue is a result of a medical problem such as anemia, which can be corrected with medication.

Little is known about the impact of exercise after diagnosis of esophageal cancer. In the absence of more definitive information, the American Cancer Society (ACS) recommends that survivors of gastrointestinal cancers follow the ACS guidelines for the prevention of cancer. The ACS guidelines on physical activity for cancer prevention follow (Brown et al, 2003).

Adopt a Physically Active Lifestyle

- Adults: Engage in at least moderate activity for 30 minutes or more on five or more days of the week; 45 minutes or more of moderate to vigorous activity on five or more days per week may further enhance reductions in the risk for breast and colon cancer.
- Children and adolescents: Engage in at least 60 minutes per day of moderate to vigorous physical activity at least five days per week.

Maintain a Healthy Weight Throughout Life

- Balance caloric intake with physical activity.
- Lose weight if currently overweight.

Bart's comment:

Exercise is always good and important for you whether you do it before treatment or during the chemotherapy and radiation protocol, and it is even strongly advisable to continue an exercise regimen during the entire recovery process. After completing the surgical procedure, the nurses will have you up and walking within minutes of having arrived from the recovery room. Exercise plays an important part in helping you stay clear of complications, especially pneumonia. An exercise regimen should be continued through the home recovery process as well. The more exercising you do, the faster you will heal, your appetite will come back sooner, and your overall condition will vastly improve.

33. What else can I do to strengthen myself before treatment?

It is important to take care of yourself before, during, and after treatment for cancer of the esophagus. Maintaining a healthy diet, getting enough rest, and using support services, if needed, can help.

Eating healthy is important whether you have a diagnosis of cancer or not. However, cancer of the esophagus may lead to problems with swallowing and a loss of appetite that make maintaining a healthy diet difficult. In fact, weight loss is one of the more common symptoms that initially bring someone to the doctor's office prior to a diagnosis of esophageal cancer. After diagnosis, it is important to maintain your weight and prevent additional weight loss. If you are having difficulty swallowing, discuss with your doctor exactly what you are able to eat and what you are not able to eat. A discussion with a dietitian may be helpful to talk about ways to increase your calories with softer or easier-to-swallow foods. In some

Feeding tube

A flexible tube passed through the nose and into the alimentary tract, through which liquid food is passed.

Gastrostomy tube (G-tube)

A type of feeding tube that is inserted directly into the stomach; this procedure is done surgically and requires sedation.

Percutaneous endoscopic gastrostomy (PEG-tube)

A type of feeding tube for those with an intact gastrointestinal tract, but unable to consume sufficient calories to meet metabolic needs; an ~30 minute procedure that requires local anesthesia.

Jejunostomy tube (J-tube)

A type of feeding tube that is placed through the skin directly into the small bowel.

cases, if weight loss is severe or if swallowing more than liquids is difficult, your doctor may recommend placing a feeding tube to help maintain your nutritional status. A **feeding tube** can be inserted through the nose into the stomach, but most often is surgically placed directly from the abdomen to the stomach. This type of tube is called a **gastrostomy tube** (or **G-tube**), a **percutaneous endoscopic gastrostomy** (**PEG-tube**), or **jejunostomy tube** (**J-tube**). This type of tube is inserted through a small incision in the abdomen during an outpatient surgical procedure. The different names indicate different placement locations within the stomach or small intestine. After placement of a feeding tube, you will be able to take meal supplements through the tube. You should also take food by mouth, if you are able.

In addition to nutrition and exercise, it is important to get adequate rest before, during, and after treatment. If you are having difficulty sleeping, exercise may help you sleep better. A diagnosis of cancer is a very stressful situation and maintaining a healthy lifestyle, including getting adequate rest, can help you to manage the stress of diagnosis and treatment.

Each person and their family will cope in different ways with a diagnosis of cancer. It is important to find a strategy that works for you and helps you to cope during this difficult time. Individuals often find that psychological support is helpful. Check with your doctor or hospital about counseling services. Psychiatrists, psychologists, and social workers can help you to develop coping strategies and gain perspectives on your situation. Social workers can also assist with more practical matters such as transportation, financial concerns, and the effects of cancer treatment on employment. Religious or spiritual counseling may also be of benefit.

During this time it is important to take care of yourself and your loved ones and not to let cancer control everything you do. This is easier said than done, but if you are having difficulty coping with your diagnosis, talk about it with your family, a dear friend, or your medical team.

Bart's comment:

Continue to eat balanced meals, exercise, and get enough rest. In effect, make yourself as strong as you can be—physically, mentally, and spiritually.

34. What are advance directives? Are a power of attorney and a living will the same thing?

Advance directive is a general term that refers to the oral and written instructions of your wishes for medical care if you are unable to speak for yourself. A medical power of attorney and a living will are both forms of advance directives. Each state regulates the use of advance directives differently. We will provide you with some general information about each of these, but you should check with your local hospital or state government (usually the Department of Health) for specifics regarding your state regulations.

A living will is a document where you can put your wishes in writing about the medical care you would like to receive in case you are unable to communicate for yourself at the end of life. State laws may limit when the living will can go into effect and may limit the treatments that apply. A living will is also called a directive to physician, declaration, or medical directive.

Advance directives

Oral and written instructions containing your wishes for medical care if you are unable to speak for yourself; includes medical power of attorney and living will.

A medical power of attorney (also called a healthcare proxy, appointment of healthcare agent, or durable power of attorney for health care) is a document that allows you to appoint someone to make decisions about your medical care. This is different from a power of attorney, which is a document that authorizes a person to make financial decisions for you and cannot be used to make healthcare decisions. You must complete a medical power of attorney in order to have someone make medical decisions for you. The person you appoint through a medical power of attorney is usually authorized to speak for you any time you are unable to make your own medical decisions, not only at the end of life.

Each document offers something the other does not, and both are important. The primary difference between a medical power of attorney and living will is that a living will does not authorize you to appoint someone to make medical decisions for you. Having both documents will help to protect your treatment decisions.

If you have questions about these documents or the specific regulations in your state, it may be helpful to talk with a social worker at the office or hospital where you are being treated.

35. So much information is available on the Internet. How do I evaluate this information to be sure that it is accurate, complete, and up-to-date?

There are more Internet sites offering health-related information every day, and it is an excellent resource for valuable health information about esophageal cancer and its treatment. However, it is important to know that there is no regulation or control of the information posted on the Internet. Many Web sites may have misleading or incorrect information. It is necessary that you distinguish good medical information from misleading or incorrect information as you look online. To do this, here are some helpful tips adapted from a National Cancer Institute fact sheet:

There is no regulation or control of the information posted on the Internet.

- Who runs the Web site?

  You must consider where the information is coming from before you consider the content. The site should clearly state who is responsible for the information. For example, a Web address ending in ".gov" denotes a federal government-sponsored site, ".org" is from a nonprofit group, and ".edu" sites are from educational institutions. Many university hospitals and comprehensive cancer centers have Web sites with searchable online patient education information. The purpose and owner of the Web site can influence what content is presented, how the content is presented, and what the site owners want to accomplish on the site. You should be wary of sites run solely by insurance or drug companies, which may be promoting their own products or services. The purpose of the site can usually be found by clicking "About This Site" on the Web page.

- Where did the information come from?

  Many Web sites post information collected from other Web sites or sources. The source of the information should be clearly stated. Ideally, medical facts and figures will have a reference to a medical journal.

- How current is the information?

  Web sites should be reviewed and updated on a regular basis—the best sites are updated every six months. Medical information can change frequently, so it is important to look for a site that has been updated recently. The most recent update or review date should be clearly noted and usually can be found at the bottom of the Web page.

- What personal information does the site collect, and why?

  Web sites routinely trace the paths visitors take through their sites to determine what pages are being used. Some sites may ask for you to subscribe or become a member. Others may charge a fee or want your personal information in order to personalize health information for you. A credible site asking for personal information should tell you exactly what they will and will not do with this information. Many commercial sites sell collected data about their users to other companies—information such as what percentage of their users has cancer, for example. In some cases they may collect and reuse information that is personally identifiable, such as your postal zip code, gender, and birth date. Be certain that you read and understand any privacy policy or similar language on the site prior to submitting any personal information. If you cannot easily find one, then do not submit any information. It is never a good idea to sign up for something you do not fully understand.

Always remember that the Internet cannot replace time with your doctor, but it can help to make you a better informed patient. Knowing what questions to ask when you see the doctor will be beneficial to getting the best health care.

CAREGIVER CONCERNS

36. Is depression a possibility?

Most people who face a diagnosis of cancer will experience a wide range of emotions from denial to despair. Your state of mind can influence all aspects of your treatment, and upon receiving a diagnosis of cancer there will need to be a period of time for adjustment and incorporation of diagnosis and treatment plans into your life. Most people are able to make this adjustment. Feelings of sadness, helplessness, and hopelessness are normal during this time. However, it is important to distinguish normal feelings of sadness and grief with a clinical depression. Clinical depression occurs when the depression is of such a magnitude that the person is unable to enjoy any of the activities that normally give them pleasure. Even though it is normal and natural to feel sad and down about a diagnosis of cancer, sometimes these feelings of sadness become so overwhelming that they take on a life of their own and become a problem in and of themselves. Patients can become so discouraged, hopeless, or full of despair that they are unable to enjoy their family or the little things in life. If you find yourself sitting at home, no longer interested in your usual activities, or withdrawing from family and friends, you may be depressed.

The good news is that most depression is treatable, and the medications are usually well tolerated with minimal side effects. The bad news is that it frequently goes undiagnosed. Several factors complicate the process of diagnosing depression in patients with cancer. The first is that many of the symptoms of depression (such as changes in eating or sleeping habits) are also symptoms associated with cancer and its treatment. Second, medical factors and some cancer treatments can cause depression. Third, patients often do not openly share emotional symptoms—a major component of the depression diagnosis—with their doctors. If you think you might be depressed, it is very important that you discuss this possibility with your doctor, who can then refer you to a psychiatrist for further evaluation and treatment.

Most frequently, patients with cancer have a type of depression called reactive depression. This is of limited duration and can be helped with counseling. Major depression is more severe and long lasting, and treatment most often includes medications such as antidepressants. When depression is treated effectively, patients experience relief of distressing symptoms and are better able to cope with their cancer and the demands of cancer treatment. Early recognition of the signs of depression will facilitate prompt diagnosis and successful treatment.

Sometimes patients are unwilling to undergo treatment for depression, thinking that it represents a sign of weakness and that they should be able to control their feelings. Nothing could be further from the truth. When you are hungry, you cannot trick your mind into thinking you are not. If you are depressed, why would you be able to trick your mind into thinking that you are not?

Bart's comment:
Every time my feelings were down, I would say to myself that God sits on my right shoulder and there is nothing that He and I together can't handle. I found post-surgery that I experienced depression somewhat, and I found that a more aggressive exercising routine brought me out of it.

37. *What is the right thing to say to my loved one?*

It is natural to feel unsure of the right things to say when someone you care about has been diagnosed with cancer, is undergoing difficult treatment, or is perhaps facing the end of his or her life. You may feel uncomfortable asking the person how he or she is doing because you are unsure of the response. You may worry that if you say the wrong thing, you will hurt him or her, or that if you talk about your own sadness, or even cry, the person will be upset. Because of your own discomfort, you may try to withdraw from the situation, distancing yourself from the person, calling less often, and putting off visits. This can result in leaving the person feeling alone at a time when he or she needs your presence more than ever before.

There is no script you can follow as a guide in knowing what to say. In fact, if you make assumptions about what the person is thinking or feeling, you may unintentionally say things that will be upsetting. The best way to start is by listening. Let the person know that if he or she would like to talk about the illness you would like to listen. At the same time, remember that not everyone communicates in the same way. Some people are very open and want to share all their thoughts and feelings. Others are more private and prefer not to talk about these things. Even for those who are generally more communicative, there may be times that he or she may feel like talking and other times when he or she doesn't. You should let the person know that you are available to listen, and should let them control when and how much they choose to share. This is a great gift that you can give.

However, listening to things that are painful or being with someone who is emotionally upset or crying may be uncomfortable. You may want to change the subject or even offer reassurances that everything will be okay, even if that may not necessarily be true. Although this may help in dealing with your own discomfort as the listener, it does not help the person speaking. In addition, it may give the message that you do not really want to hear what he or she has to say. Try to overcome your own discomfort and remain to hear what he or she is saying. It is okay to tell the person that this is difficult for you and that you are not sure how to respond to what is being said.

We often leave a great deal unsaid in an attempt to protect those we love. Yet in fact, it is the unsaid things that are often the most important to say.

You may want to speak to the person who is ill about thoughts or feelings that you are having. You may want to tell him or her about your love and concern, or of your own sadness or feelings of helplessness. You may want to try to resolve previous conflicts. You may want to talk with him or her about your own worries and concerns related to the illness. We often leave a great deal unsaid in an attempt to protect those we love. Yet in fact, it is the unsaid things that are often the most important to say.

Bart's comment:

Because some people were calling constantly to find out how I was doing and I had to ask when was the last time we spoke to get a starting point for the conversation, Ginny, my wife, and I decided to create an email network. Each week I would send an email to those who wanted to know how I was doing, and during my surgery Ginny would provide daily updates. We started with 4 people in the network, and by the time we came home from the hospital the network had grown to 85 people. We were sending emails to Europe and Australia as well as to our friends and family here in the U.S.

38. As a caregiver, how do I take care of myself during this difficult time?

Communication is very important during this time. Including your loved one in decisions will help you both cope during this difficult time. If you feel you need help, ask for it. Often, family and friends want to help but may not know how or what you need. While some may not help as you would like, others will provide significant support. Here are some tips when asking for help from family and friends:

- Identify areas where you need help, and make a list or note them on a calendar.

- Ask family and friends about when they are available and what jobs they feel most comfortable doing. You may also contact a person with a specific request, being as clear as possible about what you need.

- As you hear back from each person, note their response on your list to ensure everything is taken care of.

There are many resources available to caregivers. Many hospitals and community agencies now have support groups or services specifically for caregivers. Talk with a nurse or social worker, or contact your local American Cancer Society for services that are available in your area.

It is important at this time that you take care of yourself in addition to taking care of your loved one. Balancing your normal day-to-day tasks, such as cleaning, work, and caring for children or grandchildren, combined with the stress of a loved one diagnosed with cancer can be challenging at best. It is important not to feel guilty or selfish if you take time for yourself. By taking time for yourself, you will be better able to take care of your loved one.

Here are some tips to help you take care of yourself during this difficult time:

- Make your own health a priority. Keep doctor appointments, get enough rest, eat properly, and exercise regularly.
- Take time for leisure activities that you enjoy.
- Organize a schedule with family and friends who are willing to help.
- If you need some time off from work, speak with your supervisor or benefits department. If your company has an Employee Assistance Program, look into the services it offers. Some offer counseling services for financial issues, stress, and depression.
- Consider joining a support group for caregivers or using counseling services.
- Respect your spiritual and religious needs, and continue them as much as possible.

Despite the demands and challenges of caring for someone who has cancer, the role of a caregiver can be fulfilling and satisfying. Communication can help to work through difficult times. Asking for help can also take some of the pressure off and allow you time to take care of yourself.

39. As a caregiver, how do I know what is normal and what is urgent, and when I should call the doctor for help?

It is important to designate one person to be a key contact for communicating medical information about your loved one to family and friends, and to contact the doctor, if necessary, to ask questions. As your loved one goes through treatment, the doctor, nurse, and other members of their medical team should alert you to expected symptoms or problems and to potentially serious problems. Before each visit with the doctor, write down your key concerns and a list of questions. You may want to ask other family members or friends if they have any questions as well. Be sure to ask your most important questions first. As you are talking with the doctor, take notes. If you don't understand something, ask for it to be explained again.

Keep important phone numbers in an easy-to-locate place, and ask your doctor for a number to call in an emergency, at night, or over the weekend. If you have questions after you leave the doctor's office, call and ask to speak with someone. They may be able to answer the question or will refer you to the doctor if necessary.

Any acute or sudden symptoms such as difficulty breathing or chest pain are an emergency and warrant a call to 911 or a visit to your local emergency room.

40. What do I need to know about this disease that will help me care for my loved one while he or she is undergoing treatment?

Your love and support are tremendously valuable at this critical time. Just knowing that there is someone with whom they can share their fears and concerns is the best gift you can give. It is very important that you also keep in mind that you, as the caregiver, will have many demands made on your time and resources. Not only will you be expected to perform your usual chores, you will often be asked to assume tasks routinely done by the patient. It will also fall on you to schedule and coordinate appointments, provide transportation, run errands, obtain medications, and so forth.

There will be times that you will feel overwhelmed. Do not hesitate to ask for and accept help from other family members and friends.

There will be times that you will feel overwhelmed. Do not hesitate to ask for and accept help from other family members and friends. Find out what resources are available in your community and whether you qualify for these services. Remember that treatment is going to take months and be a major disruption of your lives. Take advantage of whatever is available to you to make the process as smooth as possible. Every family is different, and each member of the family may react to this health crisis of a loved one in different ways. Being honest about what is happening with the loved one and talking about the treatment plan are important (keeping in mind age-appropriate communication styles with young children and adolescents). But this is only one side of the picture. For many families, this is an important opportunity to create one-on-one time and family experiences outside of the boundaries of the cancer. Such things as visiting a museum, flying kites, doing community projects, simply walking together, or continuing regular enjoyable family activities as much as possible can help the family as well as you, the caregiver. Your social worker can provide individual and family counseling services, as well as group counseling and suggestions for community resources and activities.

PART FIVE

Treatment Options

What things should I consider when
making treatment choices?

Will I have pain? What are my options
to treat it if I do?

What are the latest developments in esophageal
cancer treatment? How do I find out about them?

More . . .

41. What things should I consider when making treatment choices?

You should feel comfortable with the doctor and medical team who will be treating you.

Before deciding on a treatment, be sure you are well informed as to your options. It is important to understand the treatment as well as why your doctor thinks it is the best option for you. You should consider other factors such as the location of the treatment center and insurance coverage for the treatment. You should also feel comfortable with the doctor and the medical team who will be treating you. This team includes the nurses, specialists, and support staff at the facility you choose.

42. Will I have pain? What are my options to treat it if I do?

Pain is uncommon in patients with early or locally advanced esophageal cancer. If you do experience pain, it is important to discuss it with your doctor or nurse. Only you know how much pain you are feeling, and good communication is the key to managing your pain. One of the first steps your doctor will take is to gather information about your pain. He or she will ask where it is occurring, how it feels, and how strong it is. A pain scale is a common way to measure how strong your pain is. Your doctor will ask you to rate your pain on a scale of 0 to 10 with 0 being no pain and 10 being the worst pain imaginable. Rating your pain on this scale will enable you and your doctors to monitor your pain and also your response to medications to treat the pain. In addition, keeping a diary of when you experience pain, the time of day, any activities you were doing, and what you did to relieve the pain will also help your medical team in managing your pain. After assessing your pain, your doctor may order some tests to determine what may be causing it.

There are many medications available to treat pain, and most of them can be taken as a pill or a liquid. For mild pain, medications such as aspirin, Tylenol, or Advil are used. More severe pain is treated with narcotics or opioids such as codeine, oxycodone, morphine, or hydromorphone. Some patients may worry that these medications are addicting, but that is very rarely the case. It is important that you are comfortable, and these medications work very well at treating cancer pain. They do have some side effects that we should note. Narcotics or opioids can cause sleepiness, nausea, or constipation. It is important that you monitor how you react to the medications before driving while taking them. Also, when taking narcotics or opioids you should monitor for constipation. Often, stool softeners or laxatives are prescribed to help minimize this. Pain that is described as a burning or tingling sensation may be nerve pain, and medications that treat depression or seizures are very good at treating this type of pain.

There are also non-medical methods to control or treat pain. Sometimes chemotherapy or radiation is used to treat tumors that may be causing pain. Also, a nerve block may help with certain types of pain. Massage therapy, music, and even a warm bath or shower may be helpful at alleviating pain.

If you have surgery, your pain will be managed both in the hospital and at home until it resolves. It is important to remember that after surgery you will need to be out of bed as much as possible to prevent complications that can occur following surgery. In this case, your doctor will work closely with you to monitor your pain so that you are comfortable enough to walk, take deep breaths, and cough, but are not too drowsy from the medication. You will also need to help your doctors and let them know

Patient-controlled analgesia (PCA)

Medication for pain that the patient can self-administer by pressing a button; after surgery while in the hospital, a small tube is inserted so the medication can be pumped into a vein.

Epidural catheter

A small tube placed under the skin through which medication can be administered to a patient, via a pump mechanism either at a low constant dose or when the patient presses a button, according to the physician's prescription.

how you are feeling. In most cases you will be given a **patient-controlled analgesia (PCA)** following your surgery. This is a method used to deliver better pain control to patients in the hospital. With a PCA, pain medicine is administered by a computerized pump either through a vein or through an **epidural catheter**. Pain medicine is programmed by the pump to be administered at a low dose continuously or when the patient presses a button. The pump is controlled so that the patient cannot receive more medication than is prescribed by the physician.

If you have pain during or after treatment, discuss it with your doctor. If you are taking medications for pain that are not working, tell your doctor or nurse. If you are unable to swallow, medications are available in other forms (such as a patch or a suppository) to help relieve the pain and make you more comfortable. Pain varies by individual but can be managed. Good communication is vital to finding out why you are having pain and working toward the best way to treat it. A good resource about pain is "Pain Control: A Guide for People with Cancer and Their Families" from the National Cancer Institute. Your doctor may have a copy of this booklet, or they are available from the NCI at 1-800-4-CANCER.

43. What are the latest developments in esophageal cancer treatment? How do I find out about them?

Many treatment studies are being researched in order to find more effective treatments for cancer of the esophagus. Researchers are constantly looking at methods to minimize side effects and improve symptoms of the disease. New medications are also being tested for their effectiveness in treating esophageal cancer. Talk with your doctor to find out about the latest research and treatments, or call the National Cancer Institute (1-800-4-CANCER) and ask for a PDQ (Physician Data Query) clinical trials search. A cancer information specialist will assist you in finding clinical trials. You can also search for clinical trials on the NCI's Web site (*http://www.cancer.gov/search/ clinicaltrials*). In order to search, you will need to know the type (esophageal) and stage of cancer. It is helpful to know the types of trials that are relevant to you (for instance, treatment, diagnostic, prevention, etc.). You will also be able to search for a specific drug, or a particular clinical trial by zip code or city that is convenient for you. Physician Data Query is the most comprehensive resource available to find cancer clinical trials. If you do search for clinical trials for esophageal cancer, bring your results with you to your physician to discuss what treatment is right for you.

44. What is a clinical trial?

Currently, there are more than 2,000 clinical trials for cancer in the United States and abroad. Clinical trials, or research studies, test new treatments for all kinds of diseases, including cancer. The overall goal of oncology clinical trials is to find better, more effective ways to treat cancer and help patients with cancer. Most often, we think of testing new drugs when we think of clinical trials, but research is also conducted on new approaches to surgery, diagnosis, radiation, or entirely new treatment methods such as gene therapy or biologic therapy.

Clinical trials are important for several reasons. First, patients who participate in clinical trials may be helped personally by the treatment they receive as part of the trial. There is no guarantee, however, that the treatments will help individual patients. New treatments may also have unknown side effects or risks. Clinical trials used to be thought of as a last resort and used only after standard treatment had failed. Today, for some types of cancer, the first treatment recommended may be in a clinical trial. Another important reason for clinical trials is that they contribute to our knowledge and treatment for cancer. If a new treatment is effective in a trial, it often becomes the new standard of care and can help many patients.

45. What are the different types of clinical trials?

There are several types of clinical trials, and it is important to understand the differences among them. Trials are classified into three phases, based on the type of question the trial is attempting to answer.

- Phase I: These trials are the first step in testing a new treatment. The goal of a Phase I trial is to determine the best method (intravenous, by mouth, or by injection) and the best dose of a medication. In addition, Phase I trials watch for side effects of new drugs or new doses of existing drugs. Because of their preliminary nature, these studies usually include only a limited number of patients who would not be helped by other, more known, treatments.

- Phase II: In these studies the goal is to determine whether the new treatment has an anticancer effect. For instance, does it shrink the tumor? These trials also test new treatments for specific cancers. Phase II trials also have risks and unknowns associated with them and involve small numbers of patients.

- Phase III: These studies compare the results of a new treatment with the results of people taking the standard treatment. These trials attempt to answer questions such as which group has better survival rates or which treatment has fewer side effects. Phase III trials often include large numbers of patients and are conducted nationwide.

When deciding to take part in a clinical trial, consider the decision with your family and close friends as well as the medical professionals caring for you. Clinical trials have potential benefits as well as potential drawbacks. Remember that taking part in a clinical trial is always voluntary and may be only one of your treatment options. Ask questions about the purpose of the study, possible risks and benefits, the schedule of care involved in the study, and insurance coverage for treatments, tests, or other procedures. Talking with your doctor and clearly understanding your options will enable you to make the best decision.

46. What follow-up will I need after treatment?

Your follow-up will depend on the treatment you received and how you responded to that treatment. Your doctor will discuss how often you need to be seen and what is involved in the follow-up visit or treatment. In most cases, your doctor will see you in the office and you will have a CAT scan every few months (see Question 20). He or she may also add a PET scan or an endoscopy periodically to check that your cancer has not recurred. If you notice any change in how you are feeling, let your doctor know so that your follow-up schedule can be adjusted.

If you notice any change in how you are feeling, let your doctor know so that your follow-up schedule can be adjusted.

47. How do I find out about complementary and alternative therapies?

Complementary medicine and alternative medicine are broad terms that describe a wide variety of therapeutic approaches that are outside the realm of conventional Western medicine. These healthcare practices are not intended to replace the current treatment prescribed by your physician and other medical professionals, but may be used in tandem. There is a growing body of scientific evidence about the effectiveness of these treatments, and physicians are frequently integrating once non-conventional approaches into their treatment plans. However, because some can interfere with your individual healing process, it is important to discuss these options with your primary physician.

Several reliable sources provide information about complementary and alternative therapies. Because of the rapidly changing state of knowledge about this area of medicine, the Internet provides the most up-to-date information. Resources with general information on complementary and alternative therapies include:

- Cancer Information Service of the National Cancer Institute
- National Center for Complementary and Alternative Medicine of the National Institutes of Health
- The Richard and Hinda Rosenthal Center for Complementary and Alternative Medicine at Columbia University
- MD Anderson Complementary/Integrative Medicine Education Resources
- Oncolink, from the University of Pennsylvania

Resources with information specifically about dietary supplements, including vitamins, minerals, and botanicals, include:

- Office of Dietary Supplements of the National Institutes of Health
- Center for Food Safety and Applied Nutrition of the U.S. Food and Drug Administration
- American Botanical Council (*http://www.herbalgram.org*)
- Supplement Watch (*http://www.supplementwatch.com*)
- Quackwatch (*http://www.quackwatch.com*)
- Memorial Sloan-Kettering Cancer Center (*http://www.mskcc.org/mskcc/html/11570.cfm*)

For scientific bibliographic citations related to particular therapies, see the following:

- National Library of Medicine (*http://www.nlm.nih.gov/nccam/camonpubmed.html*)

TREATMENT OPTIONS

48. How is cancer of the esophagus treated?

There are treatment options for all patients with esophageal cancer. Three kinds of treatment are used: surgery, chemotherapy, and radiation therapy. We will discuss each of these in more detail in this section. Briefly, surgery is the removal of the cancer during an operation, chemotherapy is the use of drugs to kill cancer cells in the body, and radiation therapy is the use of high-dose x-rays to kill cancer cells.

Treatment recommendations are based primarily on two factors: the extent of the disease (or stage) and the general health of the patient. The extent of disease is determined by staging tests such as CAT scans, endoscopy, and PET scans (see Questions 20 through 22 for more information on these tests and staging). The general health of the patient is determined by the doctor based on previous health conditions and tests such as heart and lung function studies.

49. What is the current standard of care for esophageal cancer?

The recommended treatment of early esophageal cancer is surgery as a single treatment. Historically, the treatment of locally advanced esophageal cancer (cancer that was not diagnosed very early but had not yet spread to other organs) was either surgery alone or radiation therapy alone. Unfortunately, neither of these treatments had good long-term results. In order to improve these results, physicians decided to try a combination of radiation and surgery. The results were better, but more work needed to be done. Chemotherapy, when used as a single treatment, has very good results for **palliation** of symptoms in a high percentage of patients. Therefore, researchers have devised strategies to combine all three modalities, and the standard of treatment continues to evolve. A number of clinical trials have been conducted to determine the effectiveness of using chemotherapy and radiation prior to surgery. More research is ongoing to improve these results, but it is generally accepted, especially in North America, that pre-operative chemotherapy and radiation therapy followed by surgery is the accepted treatment choice for locally advanced esophageal cancer.

Palliation
Used to reduce the severity or relieve the pain of a disease or symptom, but is not a cure of the underlying condition.

Bart's comment:

I had a stage III tumor which warranted chemotherapy, radiation therapy in the initial phases of my treatment, and then surgery.

50. How do I decide which treatment is best for me?

There is a lot for you to consider when choosing the best way to treat your cancer.

At this point, your test results have been reviewed by a diagnostic team of specialists, and you know the diagnosis and stage of your esophageal cancer. You may have also obtained a second opinion about your diagnosis. Based upon the expertise and recommendations of the diagnostic team of healthcare professionals, your doctor has suggested a few treatment options and developed a proposed treatment plan for what he or she believes will be the best individual treatment for you. It is important to talk with your doctor about the recommended treatment as well as any anticipated side effects of this treatment.

You have read the literature provided by your physician as well as the recommended Web sites on the Internet. You have also discussed these options with your family and/or primary caregiver. Those who are spiritual have prayed for help and health, and perhaps asked others to pray for you.

For most patients, the best treatment plan will be obvious. Expert opinion from the treatment team will align with your primary physician's recommendation, a review of the literature, and your personal wishes. Some patients, however, need a bit more time to continue their research, or to be still and think about their options before coming to a decision. Ultimately, whatever the treatment plan you decide upon, be confident that it will be the right one for you.

Bart's comment:

When I heard I had cancer I was shocked to the point of not caring or wanting to be in control. I simply wanted the doctors to do what they thought they needed to do. I found that this is not the right way to go but rather to remain in control of what is being done and take an active position in the decision process. Your team of medical experts will need to explain to you why they are suggesting this course of treatment, and you need to evaluate it and determine if it is right for you. The most important part of the project is that you totally buy into the decision because your state of mind, body, and spirit will play a major role in the outcome.

51. What is the difference between local and systemic treatment?

There are two different approaches to the treatment of cancer: local treatment and systemic treatment. Local treatment refers to the treatment of the original tumor. Systemic treatment refers to treatment that is directed at the entire body to treat any cells that may have left the original tumor site.

In most cases, surgery is considered a local treatment because it is aimed at treating the original site of the tumor. Radiation therapy is often used as a local treatment as well. Chemotherapy is considered a systemic treatment because it is given through your blood system and goes to your entire body.

SYSTEMIC TREATMENT: MEDICAL TREATMENT (DRUG THERAPY)

52. What are the current medical treatments for esophageal cancer?

The standard medical treatments for esophageal cancer are chemotherapy and radiation alone, or a combination of chemotherapy and radiation followed by surgery. The combination of chemotherapy and radiation may reduce the risk of distant recurrence of disease. The most aggressive approach to treatment combines chemotherapy and radiation followed by surgery. In about 60% to 70% of patients treated with chemotherapy and radiation, their tumor shrinks or is down-staged. This means their disease is at a lower stage than prior to when they received treatment. About 80% to 90% of these patients are then able to have surgery following chemotherapy and radiation. This still means that 10% to 20% of patients are not able to have their cancer removed following this treatment, either due to local extent of the cancer or because it has spread to other parts of the body. More research is being conducted to identify combinations of treatment regimens that will provide better results.

The most aggressive approach to treatment combines chemotherapy and radiation followed by surgery.

Bart's comment:

In my case, the stage III tumor in my esophagus was reduced in size considerably by the chemotherapy and radiation therapy that I took prior to my surgery. When the tumor was taken out by my surgeon and sent out for biopsy, it was determined that it was an early stage tumor, which was the best news I could have received.

53. What is chemotherapy?

Chemotherapy is the use of drugs to kill cancer cells. Most often the drugs are given into a vein (**intravenously**) or by mouth. Chemotherapy drugs are also called **cytotoxic drugs**; that is, they are cell-destroying medications.

Many different types of chemotherapeutic drugs exist that affect cancer cells in different ways by altering or interfering with different parts of the cell cycle. Drugs are often given in combination to try and achieve better control of the cancer.

Chemotherapy works by stopping cancer cells from growing and dividing, and chemotherapy drugs affect rapidly dividing cells in the body, including cancer cells. Side effects occur from chemotherapy partly because healthy cells can also be harmed by chemotherapy. In addition, some chemotherapy agents have other side effects that are specific to that drug or class of drugs. Side effects of chemotherapy are related to the dose and frequency of administration of the drugs as well as to characteristics of the patient. Medication is sometimes required to minimize or counteract the side effects of chemotherapy. Question 54 discusses the most common chemotherapy drugs and their side effects.

54. What are the most common drugs given?

Different drugs are given, and the choice depends on the kind of cancer you have, the stage of the disease, and your general overall health. Some of the more common agents used to treat esophageal cancer are listed in this question. Ask your nurse about more specific information for the medications used for your treatment.

Intravenously

Injection or infusion of liquid, usually medication, directly through the skin into a vein.

Cytotoxic drugs

A type of pharmaceutical substance that is detrimental or destructive to cells.

Cisplatin (Platinol)—prevents cancer cells from growing by interfering with DNA, the genetic material in cells. It is given intravenously.

Immediate Side Effects (beginning within 24 hours):

- Nausea or vomiting can begin within two hours after you have received cisplatin and last about 24 hours. Nausea may continue or recur for several days.
- Loss of appetite may occur 24 to 48 hours after treatment.
- Allergic reactions can occur, but are rare.

Early Side Effects (beginning within one week):

- Diarrhea may occur, but usually subsides within a day.
- Kidney damage may occur unless cisplatin is given with large amounts of intravenous and oral fluids.
- A ringing or "stuffy" sensation in the ears or difficulty hearing may occur within one week after treatment and may persist. The "stuffy" sensation usually subsides in two to three weeks.

Late Side Effects (beginning after one week):

- A temporary decrease in blood cell counts—red blood cells, white blood cells, and platelets—may occur 7 to 14 days after treatment. This is usually mild.
- Temporary thinning or loss of hair may occur several weeks after treatment.
- Numbness, tingling, or burning in the hands or feet may occur after several treatments, but is uncommon.
- This medication may have temporary or permanent effects on your hearing, such as ringing or a stuffy sensation in the ears, hearing loss of high frequency sounds, and difficulty hearing when there is background noise. Discuss any change in your hearing with your doctor.

Special Points:
- Drink fluids as instructed by your doctor.
- Take your antinausea medication as instructed.
- Do not take aspirin, ibuprofen (e.g., Motrin, Advil), products containing them, or similar products unless your doctor prescribes them. (Ask your doctor or nurse for a complete list of NSAIDs and products containing aspirin, or ask your pharmacist for a list.)
- Tell your doctor or nurse if you are taking any other medications, including over-the-counter preparations that do not require a prescription, herbal remedies, vitamins, or dietary supplements. Some of these may interfere with your chemotherapy.

Call Your Doctor or Nurse If You:
- Are urinating less frequently than usual or in small amounts.
- Have excessive nausea, vomiting, or diarrhea and are unable to eat or drink for more than 24 hours after receiving the drug.
- Have a fever of 100.5°F (38°C) or higher.
- Have black bowel movements, bruising, a faint red rash, or any other signs of bleeding.
- Have any unexpected, unexplained problems.
- Have any questions or concerns.

5-FU (Fluorouracil, Adrucil)—interferes with an enzyme that cancer cells need to live and grow. It is given intravenously.

Early Side Effects (beginning within one week):

- Mild nausea and vomiting may occur while you take this drug.
- You may experience diarrhea with this medication.
- You may develop soreness in the mouth.

Late Side Effects (beginning after one week):

- A temporary decrease in blood cell counts—white blood cells and platelets—may occur one to two weeks after treatment.
- Dryness and scaling of the nails, cuticles, and skin of the hands may occur four to six weeks after treatment.
- Darkening of the nail beds, the skin, and the veins in which the drug was given may begin four to six weeks after receiving the drug and may persist.
- Temporary thinning of the hair may occur three to four weeks after each treatment.
- Nasal stuffiness and watering of the eyes may occur three to four weeks after treatment.

Special Points:

- Do not take aspirin, ibuprofen (e.g., Motrin, Advil), products containing them, or similar products unless your doctor prescribes them. (Ask your doctor or nurse for a complete list of NSAIDs and products containing aspirin, or ask your pharmacist for a list.)
- Protect your skin from overexposure to the sun. Wear protective clothing and use a sunscreen with a sun protection factor (SPF) of 15 or greater when in the sun.

- Tell your doctor or nurse if you are taking any other medications, including over-the-counter preparations that do not require a prescription, herbal remedies, vitamins, or dietary supplements. Some of these may interfere with your chemotherapy.

Call Your Doctor or Nurse If You:
- Have a fever of 100.5°F (38°C) or higher.
- Have more than three loose bowel movements a day over your normal bowel routine.
- Have black bowel movements, bruising, faint red rash, or any other signs of bleeding.
- Develop mouth sores.
- Have any unexpected or unexplained problems.
- Have any question or concerns.

Irinotecan (Camptosar, CPT-11)—is a partly manmade drug derived from an extract of a plant that grows in Asia. It kills cancer cells by interfering with an enzyme that helps DNA unwind so that cells can reproduce. It is given intravenously.

Immediate Side Effects (beginning within 24 hours):
- Abdominal cramping can occur while the drug is being given.
- Mild sweating, with or without feeling warm, can occur while the drug is given.
- You may experience nausea and vomiting.
- Diarrhea may occur with this medication.

Early Side Effects (beginning within one week):
- You may experience a runny nose.

Late Side Effects (beginning after one week):

- A temporary decrease in white blood cell count (cells that help fight infection) can develop.
- Possible temporary thinning or loss of hair can occur.
- Diarrhea can occur after the second or third cycle of treatment.
- You may experience fatigue.

Special Points:

- Diarrhea that occurs during or within a few hours of treatment usually goes away by itself. Do not take Imodium (loperamide) under these circumstances, as it can lead to constipation.
- If diarrhea occurs other than on the day of treatment, begin taking Imodium when diarrhea starts. Although the package cautions not to take this amount, take two Imodium tablets at the first sign of diarrhea. Then take 1 tablet every 2 hours (or 2 tablets every 4 hours at night) until you have gone 12 hours without diarrhea. If Imodium is not effective after 36 hours, call your physician.
- Do not take aspirin, ibuprofen (e.g., Motrin, Advil), products containing them, or similar products unless your doctor prescribes them. (Ask your doctor or nurse for a complete list of NSAIDs and products containing aspirin, or ask your pharmacist for a list.)
- Tell your doctor or nurse if you are taking any other medications, including over-the-counter preparations that do not require a prescription, herbal remedies, vitamins, or dietary supplements. Some of these may interfere with your chemotherapy.

Call Your Doctor or Nurse If You Have:

- A fever of 100.5° F (38° C) or higher.
- Black bowel movements, bruising, faint red rash, or other signs of bleeding.
- Diarrhea of any sort, including an increase in frequency of bowel movements.
- Any unexpected, unexplained problems.
- Any questions or concerns.

Paclitaxel (Taxol)—works by interfering with the cancer cell's ability to grow. It is given intravenously.

Early Side Effects:

- In rare circumstances, patients may develop an allergic reaction with a rash, facial flushing, or have trouble breathing. Benadryl (diphenhydramine), Decadron (dexamethasone), and Zantac (ranitidine) are given before paclitaxel to help prevent this reaction.
- Mild nausea and vomiting, though uncommon, may occur while you are taking paclitaxel.
- Fatigue can occur during treatment.
- Joint pain and body aches may occur and can usually be relieved by acetaminophen (e.g., Tylenol).

Late Side Effects:

- Mouth sores may develop within four to seven days.
- Hair thinning or loss may occur, depending on your treatment schedule.
- Numbness and tingling in the hands and feet may occur.
- A temporary decrease in blood cell counts—especially white blood cell counts—may occur about one week after treatment.

Special Points:

- Tell your doctor if you are also taking ketoconazole (Nizoral).
- You or your partner should not get pregnant while you are taking paclitaxel. You must use an effective contraceptive during treatment.
- Speak with your doctor before you get any vaccine (e.g., a flu shot).
- Check with your doctor or pharmacist before you take any prescribed or over-the-counter medicine, herbal remedy, or vitamin supplement, because some can interfere with your chemotherapy treatment.
- Do not take aspirin, ibuprofen (e.g., Motrin, Advil), products containing them, or similar products unless your doctor prescribes them. (Ask your doctor or nurse for a complete list of NSAIDs and products containing aspirin, or ask your pharmacist for a list.)
- You must not breastfeed during your treatment.

Call Your Doctor or Nurse If You:

- Develop a fever higher than 100.5° F (38.0° C).
- Develop mouth sores that prevent you from eating or drinking.
- Have joint aches or pain not controlled by Tylenol (acetaminophen).
- Have uncontrolled nausea or diarrhea.
- Have pain in your back.
- Have any unexpected or unexplained problems.
- Have any questions or concerns.

Docetaxel (Taxotere)—works by interfering with the cancer cell's ability to multiply and grow. It is given intravenously.

Immediate Side Effects (beginning within 24 hours):
- Flushing of the skin, chest tightness, shortness of breath, and back discomfort may occur occasionally during the infusion. These symptoms disappear when the infusion is stopped. A medication will be prescribed to prevent these symptoms before you receive docetaxel.

Early Side Effects (beginning within one week):
- A temporary decrease in blood cell counts, particularly white blood cell counts, may occur within one week of treatment.
- A red, raised, itchy rash; peeling of the skin on hands and feet; and ridging and splitting of fingernails and toenails may occur after any dose.
- Redness or swelling may occur at the injection site.

Late Side Effects (beginning after one week):
- Temporary thinning or loss of hair may begin two to three weeks after treatment.
- Swelling of arms and legs, bloating, and weight gain may occur after receiving docetaxel for several months. Fluid can also accumulate around the lungs or in the abdominal cavity.
- Numbness, tingling of fingers and/or toes, or both may also occur after receiving docetaxel many times.
- Epiphora (excessive tearing caused by a narrowing of the first portion of the tear ducts) is a recently reported symptom of taxotere. It is seen more often when patients receive weekly doses of taxotere.

Special Points:

- Before receiving docetaxel, you will be given a prescription for a medication to prevent side effects. The nurse will review with you the schedule for taking this medication. Please inform the nurse if you are unable to take the medication as ordered.

- Do not take aspirin, ibuprofen (e.g., Motrin, Advil), products containing them, or similar products unless your doctor prescribes them. (Ask your doctor or nurse for a complete list of NSAIDs and products containing aspirin, or ask your pharmacist for a list.)

- Tell your doctor or nurse if you are taking any other medications, including over-the-counter preparations that do not require a prescription, herbal remedies, vitamins, or dietary supplements. Some of these may interfere with your chemotherapy.

- You may need to have periodic ophthalmologic evaluations to monitor for epiphora. If you do develop this symptom, an ophthalmologist can treat it by surgically inserting **stents** to keep the tear duct open.

Call Your Doctor or Nurse If You Have:

- Shortness of breath.
- Difficulty swallowing.
- Pain, redness, swelling, or blistering near the injection site.
- Nausea or vomiting and are unable to eat or drink.
- A fever of 100.5°F (38°C) or higher.
- Swelling of the arms or legs.
- Excessive tearing of your eye(s).
- Any unexpected, unexplained problems.
- Any questions or concerns.

Stent

A thread, rod, or catheter that is inserted into the cell wall of the esophagus to keep it open.

Mitomycin (Mutamycin)—stops cancer cells from growing by interfering with DNA, the genetic material in cells.

Immediate Side Effects (beginning within 24 hours):
- Nausea and vomiting are unusual, but may begin several hours after treatment and last for several hours.

Early Side Effects (beginning within one week):
- Mouth sores can begin five to seven days after treatment.

Late Side Effects (beginning after one week):
- A temporary decrease in blood cell counts—red blood cells, white blood cells, and platelets—can occur two to three weeks after treatment. The platelet count can remain low for several weeks.
- A temporary thinning or loss of hair can begin two to three weeks after each treatment.
- Damage to lung tissue resulting in shortness of breath can occur after several doses.

Special Points:
- Do not take aspirin, ibuprofen (e.g., Motrin, Advil), products containing them, or similar products unless your doctor prescribes them. (Ask your doctor or nurse for a complete list of NSAIDs and products containing aspirin, or ask your pharmacist for a list.)
- Tell your doctor or nurse if you are taking any other medications, including over-the-counter preparations that do not require a prescription, herbal remedies, vitamins, or dietary supplements. Some of these may interfere with your chemotherapy.

Call Your Doctor or Nurse If You:

- Experience shortness of breath.
- Experience pain, redness, swelling, or blistering at or near the injection site.
- Have excessive vomiting and are unable to eat or drink for more than 24 hours after treatment.
- Have a fever of 100.5° F (38° C) or higher.
- Have black bowel movements, bruising, faint red rash, or any other signs of bleeding.
- Develop mouth sores or a sore throat.
- Have any unexpected, unexplained problems.
- Have any questions or concerns.

Oxaliplatin (Eloxatin)—works by inhibiting DNA synthesis and is a platinum-based chemotherapy drug in the same family as cisplatin and carboplatin.

Early Side Effects (beginning within one week):

- Sensitivity to cold when handling cold objects, which can last for a few days or longer after treatment.
- Tightness or painful sensation in the throat, caused by cold temperatures.
- An allergic reaction is rare.
- Nausea or vomiting.
- Diarrhea.

Late Side Effects (beginning after one week):

- A temporary decrease in the blood cells that help fight infection (white blood cells).
- Fatigue.
- Nausea and vomiting.
- Numbness, tingling, or burning in the fingers or toes.

Special Points:
- If you are being treated on cold winter days, carry a scarf to breathe through.
- Tell your doctor or nurse if you are taking any other medicines or have changed your medicines.
- Take your antinausea medication the way your nurse instructed you.
- Avoid aspirin, NSAIDs, and vitamin E, which can add to bleeding problems. Ask your doctor before you take them.
- Try not to go out in the cold or drink cold fluids.

Call Your Doctor or Nurse If You:
- Have a fever of 100.5° F (38° C) or higher.
- Have black bowel movements, bruising, faint red rash, or any other signs of bleeding.
- Are unable to eat or drink for more than one day.
- Have any unexpected, unexplained problems.
- Have any questions or concerns.

Capecitabine (Xeloda)—an oral chemotherapy medication that is converted to 5-fluorouracil in the tumor where it inhibits DNA synthesis and slows growth of tumor tissue.

Early Side Effects (beginning within one week):
- Nausea and vomiting.
- Diarrhea, which can be severe.
- Mouth sores.
- Loss of appetite.
- Abdominal pain.
- Fatigue.
- Swelling in your hands and feet.
- Heart damage, which is very rare.

Late Side Effects (beginning after one week):

- A temporary decrease in blood cell counts two to three weeks after treatment. White blood cells and platelets are mostly affected.
- A change in liver function. It usually returns to normal when the drug is stopped.
- A skin rash or tingling sensation on the hands and feet.

Special Points:

- This medication can be damaging to an unborn child. Ask your doctor or nurse about the type of birth control you should use. Tell your doctor immediately if you think you or your partner might be pregnant.
- Speak to your doctor before you get any vaccines, such as the flu vaccine.
- Tell your doctor or nurse if you are taking any other medicines or have changed your medicines.
- Take your antidiarrhea medication the way your nurse instructed you.
- Avoid aspirin, NSAIDs, and vitamin E, which can add to bleeding problems. Ask your doctor before you take them.
- Follow your doctor's or nurse's instructions on how to care for your mouth.

Call Your Doctor or Nurse If You:

- Have diarrhea that is frequent or doesn't get better.
- Have nausea that is frequent or doesn't get better.
- Have any sign of bleeding, including black bowel movements, bruising, faint red rash.
- Develop mouth sores.
- Develop tingling on your hands and feet.
- Have unexplained weight gain or swelling in the hands or feet.

- Have a fever of 100.5° F (38° C) or higher.
- Have any questions or concerns.

55. Are chemotherapy and radiation given before or after surgery?

Chemotherapy and radiation can be given either before or after surgery. **Adjuvant therapy** is treatment given after surgery to lessen your chances that the cancer will return. **Neoadjuvant therapy** is the same type of treatment, except that it is given before surgery.

Physicians differ on their preference for treatment, and past research has not found a clear benefit for one treatment over another. A slight survival advantage has been reported when chemotherapy and radiation are given before surgery. It is thought this may relieve symptoms such as dysphagia and increase the chances of complete removal of the tumor at the time of surgery. Neither option has proven to be clearly superior. Research is ongoing to identify the best schedule of treatment.

Discuss each of these options with your physician to better understand the benefits and drawbacks of each approach.

Bart's comment:

I had chemotherapy and radiation therapy first and then surgery. For me that was the proper protocol in my case, as evidenced by the results I have had since surgery.

Adjuvant therapy

Chemotherapy given after surgery to lessen the chances that cancer will recur.

Neoadjuvant therapy

Chemotherapy given before surgery to shrink or isolate the tumor.

56. When would someone need chemotherapy?

Surgery is recommended as a single treatment for patients with Stage I or early Stage II esophageal cancer. Chemotherapy is recommended for patients with Stage II disease or higher. The advantage of chemotherapy is that it travels throughout the entire body and, potentially, may kill cancer cells that have spread beyond the original tumor site. Additionally, when chemotherapy is combined with radiation, more cancer cells are killed. Chemotherapy should be included in the treatment plan for all patients with esophageal cancer that was not found at a very early stage.

57. What is radiation therapy?

Radiation therapy uses x-rays to kill cancer cells and shrink tumors. Radiation is like surgery in that it is a localized type of treatment that affects defined areas in the body, and it is different from chemotherapy, which circulates throughout the body. Radiation can come from a machine outside the body, which is called **external beam radiation therapy**. It also can be delivered directly to the tumor in a treatment called **brachytherapy**. External beam radiation is the most common type of radiation used to treat cancer of the esophagus. External beam radiation is usually delivered daily, Monday to Friday. A treatment course, depending on the area being treated and on the size of the cancer, can be anywhere from 5–10 treatments to 28–35 treatments. Very specific targets are marked on your body, using complicated CAT scanning to determine the exact area to be treated. This process (called **simulation**) can take several hours. From there, medical physicists and the radiation oncologist plan the total dose of the radiation, the number of

External beam radiation therapy

A type of x-ray therapy that comes from a machine outside of the body, usually delivered daily in a specific series of treatments.

Brachytherapy

A type of radiation therapy where a source of irradiation (such as radioactive seeds) is implanted directly into or near the tumor permanently or for a specified time.

Simulation

A process in which specific areas on the cancer patient's body are marked, sometimes using computed tomography, in preparation for targeting the tumor(s) with radiation therapy.

treatments, and the field size. Usually, a couple of days before beginning radiation you will undergo a "beam check" to ensure that the radiation prescription is exact and appropriate. Each daily radiation treatment takes approximately 10 minutes.

58. Is radiation a recommended treatment for esophageal cancer?

Radiation as a single treatment for esophageal cancer is not effective for a curative approach. Instead, it is combined with chemotherapy so that the radiation provides local control (to the area of the primary tumor) and the chemotherapy provides systemic control (from spread of the cancer through the blood or lymph systems).

Radiation is also used as a palliative treatment to relieve symptoms such as difficulty swallowing, pain, or other symptoms.

MEDICAL TREATMENT: SIDE EFFECTS

59. What are the common side effects of chemotherapy and radiation? Are these side effects temporary or permanent?

Chemotherapy works by targeting the rapidly dividing cells in the body. Cancer cells divide rapidly, but many beneficial cells in the body also divide rapidly and are negatively affected by chemotherapy. The lining of the digestive tract is affected, which can lead to nausea, vomiting, diarrhea, poor appetite, and sores in the mouth. Hair cells divide rapidly, so chemotherapy can lead to loss of hair. The body's blood cells divide rapidly, so chemotherapy can lead to anemia, reduced blood clotting ability, and decreased ability to fight an infection. Medications and treatments can lessen the intensity of these side effects, and the occurrence of the side effects varies based on the general health of the patient and dose of the drug given. These side effects usually go away gradually after treatment stops. Some drugs may have longer-term side effects. An example of one is cisplatin, which can have temporary or permanent effects on hearing. If you have hearing loss prior to treatment, your doctor may recommend a different drug or may monitor you closely for hearing changes during treatment.

Radiation works by using x-rays to kill cancer cells. The x-rays are aimed at the part of the body with the tumor to kill cancer cells while minimizing damage to surrounding healthy tissue. When being treated with external radiation therapy, the patient is not radioactive, so no special precautions are necessary. Radiation therapy can lead to fatigue or feelings of tiredness as treatment progresses. It can also cause skin problems to the area being treated, an upset stomach, diarrhea, difficulty swallowing, and a cough. These side effects may worsen as treatment progresses. Radiation continues to work even after the treatment has finished. Side effects, therefore, may take some time to resolve, but do gradually improve following treatment.

60. How can side effects be treated?

Some general side effects of both radiation and chemotherapy are listed next with suggestions to help manage them. As always, discuss any side effects you may be having with your doctor or nurse who can help you manage them.

- Fatigue: a feeling of tiredness or lack of energy that is a common side effect of chemotherapy and radiation. The exact cause is not known and may be related to a variety of factors. Rest does not always relieve this type of fatigue. Some suggestions to help manage fatigue include planning rest periods during the day and taking short breaks or naps instead of one long rest. Continue to do the activities you enjoy but at easier levels or for shorter periods of time. Short walks or light exercise have been found to help with fatigue. Eating well and drinking plenty of fluids may help with fatigue.

- Nausea and vomiting: frequent side effects of chemotherapy that are seen less frequently with radiation therapy. New drugs are available to help prevent nausea and vomiting and help to make them less severe when they do occur. If you do experience nausea or vomiting, discuss it with your doctor or nurse, especially if you are unable to keep liquids or medications down. Some suggestions to help manage nausea and vomiting include eating small meals instead of larger ones and chewing food well for easier digestion. Drink liquids at least an hour before or after meals, instead of with meals, and drink frequently in small amounts. Eating foods cold or at room temperature can help if strong smells bother you. Drinking decaffeinated sodas that have lost their fizz may also help.

- Hair loss: a common side effect of chemotherapy, but it does not occur with all drugs. Discuss this with your doctor if you are at risk for this side effect. When hair loss does occur, it can become thinner or may fall out completely and occur on all body parts. The hair usually grows back once the treatment is over and may grow back a different color or texture.

- Anemia: caused by a decrease in red blood cells' ability to carry enough oxygen. Anemia may lead to feelings of shortness of breath, tiredness, and weakness. Your doctor will check your blood counts frequently during treatment. Medications are available to help boost the growth of red blood cells in your body. If your blood count falls too low, you may need a blood transfusion to help raise the number of red blood cells in your body.

- Low white blood cell count: can lead to being at higher risk for an infection. White blood cells help our body fight off infections. These cells divide rapidly and may be destroyed by chemotherapy. Your doctor will check your blood counts regularly during treatment and will be able to tell you if you are at risk for an infection. Medications are available to help speed the recovery of white blood cells and can greatly lower the risk of serious infection. Several simple steps can help to prevent an infection: Washing your hands before you eat and after using the bathroom will help. Avoid standing water, for example, from flower pots, or vases of cut flowers, or humidifiers. Wear gloves when gardening or cleaning up. Do not eat any raw fish, seafood, meat, or eggs. Stay away from anyone you know who is actively sick or has the flu, chicken pox, or a fever. Call your doctor immediately if you experience a temperature over 100° F, chills, sore throat, cough, or burning on urination.

- Low platelet counts: Platelets are a type of blood cell that help your blood to clot. If your platelets are low, you will be at risk to bleed and will bruise more easily. Your doctor will check your platelet count frequently during treatment and will alert you if you are at risk for bleeding. If your platelet count

Your doctor will check your blood counts regularly during treatment and will be able to tell you if you are at risk for an infection.

gets too low, you can receive a platelet transfusion to replace some of your platelets. There are also medications that can help increase your platelets. If you do have a low platelet count, you will need to avoid behaviors or activities that may cause bleeding or bruising. Some of these include using a soft toothbrush, blowing your nose gently, avoiding activities that may result in injury, and using an electric shaver instead of a razor.

- Mouth sores: sores in the mouth or throat are called stomatitis or mucositis. Mouth sores can be painful and may become infected. Some steps to help prevent or minimize mouth sores involve practicing good oral hygiene. Brush your teeth after every meal and before going to bed. Avoid mouthwashes with alcohol, as they may be irritating to the oral mucosa. Your doctor or nurse can recommend a non-irritating, gentle mouthwash that will help. If you do develop mouth sores, avoid irritating or acidic foods such as orange juice or tomatoes, spicy foods, or dry, coarse foods such as crackers, popcorn, and raw vegetables. Foods that are cold or room temperature are usually more soothing than hot foods.

- Skin irritation: radiation can often cause irritation of the skin that is being treated. This area can often become red or dry. Do not expose this area to the sun, and avoid wearing clothes that rub the area. Your radiation oncologist or nurse will recommend a soap or lotion that you should use. Do not use any lotions or soap without checking first.

61. What happens if I don't have side effects? Is the treatment working?

Medications have been developed to help manage the side effects of chemotherapy. Today, we have medications to help with nausea and vomiting, decreased blood counts, and other side effects of chemotherapy. In addition, side effects of both chemotherapy and radiation tend to be cumulative and may get worse as someone has had more treatment.

If you do not have side effects, don't worry. Continue to take care of yourself by eating well and getting some exercise. Your doctor is managing your treatment well and is preventing any side effects. The only way to tell if the treatment is working is to repeat CAT scans or other staging procedures after several cycles of chemotherapy and radiation to assess how your cancer has changed.

Bart's comment:

In my case I did not have any side effects from the chemo and radiation protocol. I was concerned and expressed that concern to my doctors. Here they were telling me of the possible side effects and nothing was happening. They reassured me that the chemotherapy and radiation therapy were working, and when we were finished with that phase of my treatment my tumor had reduced in size considerably.

If you do not have side effects, don't worry— your doctor is managing your treatment well and is preventing any side effects.

MEDICAL TREATMENT: SURGERY

62. What is an esophagectomy?

Esophagectomy

The surgical removal of part or most of the diseased esophagus and part of the stomach, followed by the rebuilding of a new esophagus using tissue from the stomach or the small or large intestine.

An **esophagectomy** is the surgical removal of part of or most of the esophagus and proximal part of the stomach. It is often the only treatment for cancer of the esophagus, especially when the cancer is in an early stage. In most cases, however, surgery is combined with chemotherapy and radiation to treat esophageal cancer.

During an esophagectomy, the surgeon removes the part of the esophagus that contains the tumor with additional length of normal esophagus and possibly part of the stomach to ensure complete removal of the cancer. The next part of the operation is to make a new esophagus, using either the stomach or part of the small or large intestine. Most surgeons prefer to use the stomach because of certain advantages: it has the most dependable blood supply, and it takes only one connection (**anastomosis**) to attach the stomach to the remaining esophagus. When the colon is used, three connection sites are necessary: one connecting to the esophagus, one to the remaining stomach, and another attaching back to the colon itself. The anastomosis is the name for the site where the remaining esophagus is connected to the "new" esophagus (see **Figure 5**).

Anastomosis

A natural communication or connection, direct or indirect, between two blood vessels or other tubular structures; the surgical connection of severed organs to form a continuous channel.

In addition to removing the tumor in the esophagus, the surgeon may remove or sample adjacent lymph nodes and tissue near the tumor. All of the tissue that is removed will be checked by a pathologist for the presence of cancer cells.

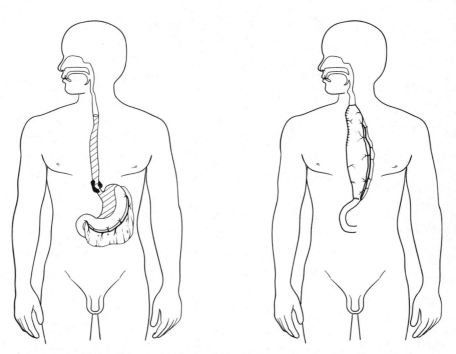

Figure 5 (Left) Normal anatomy (striped area is removed at the time of resection). (Right) Reconstruction of the esophagus and repositioning of the stomach.

An esophagectomy is a major surgical procedure that carries potential risks, complications, and mortality. Surgeons with training in thoracic or gastrointestinal surgery have experience performing this operation, and in some hospitals the two will work together, with the thoracic surgeon doing the chest part of the operation while a gastric surgeon will do the abdominal part of the operation. Recently, some studies have found that patients undergoing major or complicated procedures such as esophageal resection at hospitals that performed a low volume of esophagectomies were at increased risk of postoperative complications and death. Therefore, it is vital to seek care at a hospital where a high volume of such procedures is being performed so that you are being treated by an experienced surgeon and his or her team.

63. What are the different types of esophagectomy?

Several techniques can be used to remove the tumor and any adjacent lymph nodes that might be involved and to reconstruct the esophagus using either the stomach or the colon or, less frequently, the small bowel (see **Figure 6** for diagrams of the surgical incisions for transhiatal and transthoracic esophagectomy).

Transhiatal esophagectomy is performed through an incision in the neck and another incision in the abdomen, extending from the lower part of the breast bone to almost the umbilicus. After the stomach is isolated, the esophagus is dissected through an opening in the diaphragm and through the incision in the neck. Most of this can be done under direct vision, but in the mid-chest, it is usually done by the surgeon using feel rather than direct vision. Surgeons call this a "blind dissection." The stomach is brought up into the neck, and the esophagus, from the neck down to the stomach, including a small rim of the stomach, is removed. The stomach is attached to the esophagus in the neck either by a stapling device or by manually suturing the two together. The advantage of this particular surgical technique is that it avoids a more painful incision in the chest where the ribs need to be spread. However, because of the "blind dissection," some of the tissues (including the lymph nodes around the esophagus) may not be widely excised. It is possible that remaining lymph nodes have cancer that later could spread to other organs in the body.

Transthoracic esophagogastrectomy is a surgical procedure started in the mid-1930s by two British surgeons that remains the gold standard of surgery for esophageal cancer. It requires an incision in the abdomen from the

---

Transhiatal esophagectomy

Surgical type of resection of the esophagus where the incision is made from the cervical section of the neck from above and up from the abdomen from below.

Transthoracic esophagogastrectomy

Surgical type of resection of the esophagus through a thoracotomy incision (breast bone to the umbilicus, plus another incision on the right side of the chest).

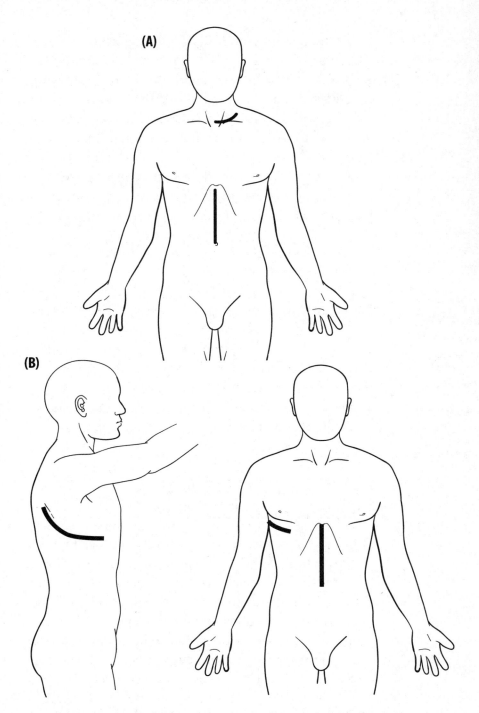

Figure 6 Surgical incisions for (A) transhiatal and (B) transthoracic esophagectomy.

breast bone to the umbilicus, plus an incision on the right side of the chest. Through the chest incision, the esophagus can be dissected with the surrounding lymph nodes and wide margins. The stomach may be attached to the esophagus in the chest if there are adequate margins next to the tumor or, for better margins, the surgeon may elect to go into the neck. The advantage of this surgical procedure is that the tumor is removed with the surrounding tissues and lymph nodes adequately. The pain associated with spreading the ribs can be effectively controlled by placing an epidural catheter, allowing the patient to control the amount of pain medication needed for satisfactory relief.

Minimally invasive surgery marks a relatively recent advance in surgical techniques and has also been applied to removal of the esophagus. A number of variations on this procedure using a number of small incisions over the abdomen and chest have been described. These techniques are new and have yet to prove themselves as far as adequacy, completeness of tumor removal, and cure rates are concerned.

64. What are the risks and complications of surgery?

An esophagectomy is a major surgical procedure and carries a number of risks. Some of the complications are the same as those which may occur after any type of surgery and others are specific to esophageal surgery. Your medical history and general overall health will impact your recovery from the operation and chances to develop a complication after surgery. We will review some of the more common risks and complications here. Your surgeon will review the risks and potential complications of your surgery with you.

Minimally invasive surgery

An operative procedure that results in the smallest possible incision or no incision at all; includes laparoscopic, laparoscopically-assisted, thoracoscopic, and endoscopic procedures.

Two of the most common complications after surgery are pneumonia and infection. An infection can occur after any surgical procedure but is minimized with good surgical procedures. The hospital staff will monitor you closely after surgery for any signs or symptoms of an infection.

Postoperative pain and limited or no activity leads to an individual taking shallow breaths. This results in parts of the lung not being fully expanded. Incompletely expanded lungs collect secretions. Just as a stagnant pool of water can grow all kinds of organisms, secretions that settle in the lung start growing bacteria and cause pneumonia. Pneumonia is the most common complication of surgery and the most common cause of the patient not surviving the operation. It can be prevented by preparing oneself prior to surgery. Aerobic exercises, such as walking for about an hour a day, will get the patient in better physical condition (see Question 33). Stopping smoking is also very important to preparing yourself for surgery (see Question 8).

After the surgery, it is important to be taking deep breaths and coughing even though you may not bring up any sputum. Coughing is the best way to re-expand your lungs and keep them expanded. Expanded lungs will not collect secretions and hence you will reduce the chances of getting pneumonia.

During preoperative teaching, the nurse will give you an **incentive spirometer** (**Figure 7**) and explain to you how it is used. An incentive spirometer is a small plastic device that you will use to inhale and expand your lungs. Just as the name implies, it induces you to take deep breaths, and you should use it frequently before and after surgery. You will also be asked to cough after walking or using the incentive spirometer in order to move any secretions that may be in your lungs.

Two of the most common complications after surgery are pneumonia and infection.

TREATMENT OPTIONS

Incentive spirometer

A device used to help the patient inhale and expand the lungs.

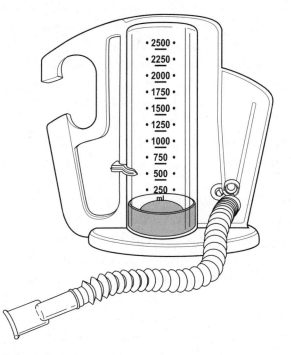

Figure 7 Incentive spirometer.

Cardiac complications are also common after surgery. Irregular heart rhythms or other heart problems can occur after a major surgery such as an esophagectomy. Depending on your age and your previous medical history, assessment of your heart is usually done before surgery. A cardiologist may examine and perform certain tests to ensure that you are able to tolerate the surgery. In some cases, medications or special monitoring may be necessary following surgery. If you have pre-existing cardiac problems, such an assessment becomes important, and a cardiologist may get involved in your care prior to and after the surgery.

Some complications are specific to the surgical procedure of an esophagectomy. One of these is an **anastomotic leak**. At the time of the operation, the stomach or the

Anastomotic leak

A condition in which the tissues have not healed completely from an esophagectomy and liquids or saliva leak into the chest cavity. To treat this condition, more time must be allowed for the tissues to heal completely or the patient undergoes further surgery.

colon is attached to the remaining esophagus with sutures or staples. Tissues have to heal to permanently seal it off. If there was a problem with healing, liquids or saliva could leak into the chest cavity. This is a rare but potentially serious complication. Your surgeon will probably not allow you to eat or drink until it heals. Treatment for an anastomotic leak includes allowing more time for the site to heal or more surgery.

65. How do I prepare for surgery?

Anyone who undergoes a surgical procedure needs to be in the best possible physical shape they can be, and this is especially true of those undergoing an esophagectomy. It is a major undertaking and a drain on one's physical reserves. Getting into the best physical condition must be the primary goal in the patient's mind. This is no less a task than an athlete getting into shape for a competition. For patients who are receiving preoperative treatment, it is very important that they develop and maintain a program of physical activity throughout the course of treatment. There will be times when feelings of fatigue will interrupt the routine, but even walking 15 to 20 minutes a day will help. There is a hiatus of four to six weeks from the end of preoperative chemotherapy and radiation to surgery. This is a good time to recuperate from the effects of treatment and restart or intensify your exercise routine.

Good mental health is as important as good physical health, and if at all possible this would be a good time to get away for a week or two. You may also find it helpful to speak with someone who has undergone the surgery and is now fully recovered. Some institutions have a patient-to-patient volunteer program, but if yours doesn't, your doctor or nurse may be able to arrange for you to speak with someone.

Bart's comment:

I exercised by walking 3 times a week prior to surgery. I would go to the mall when the weather was bad and walk around the mall at 7:00 AM. It was open and there were other people there exercising as I was, so I did not feel out of place.

66. What is the hospital stay like?

Unless there is a specific reason for early admission, patients are admitted on the same day as the surgery. The average hospital stay is 10 to 14 days. During surgery, some tubes and drains may be placed to drain fluid from the stomach and/or chest. The different types of tubes and drains you will need depend on the type of surgery your physician performs. Your doctor and nurse will have spoken to you beforehand about the tubes you should expect. Most surgeons will obtain a barium swallow after about a week to check on the healing of the anastomosis. The barium swallow will tell your surgeon if the anastomosis is healed. If the barium swallow looks normal, you will be started on sips of clear liquids, and your diet will be slowly advanced until you are able to eat regular food. It is also at this time that your tubes and drains are removed. It is rare that someone will be discharged with any drainage tubes.

Bart's comment:

I was in the hospital for 10 days and my recovery went without any complications. They had me up and walking the day after my surgery, and I did about 1 mile a day as exercise. The exercise, so important prior to the surgery, was emphasized even more during my hospital stay. In addition to walking, I did breathing and coughing exercises as well, all aimed at avoiding lung infections.

67. What is the success rate for surgery?

Nationally, about a third of patients having esophagectomies will develop some minor complications. However, in about 5% of patients undergoing esophagectomy, the complications are fatal. In a center with expertise in this disease and the procedure, the mortality rate for surgery may be half of that percentage. Addition of chemotherapy and radiation as a multimodality treatment has also enabled more patients to undergo surgery and has not increased the complications of surgery.

Bart's comment:

The key to a more successful outcome is selecting a hospital and surgeon that have done this procedure numerous times over the last six months. The attention a hospital pays to the recovery process is very important. A patient should tour the hospital facility that they are considering to see how patients are cared for in the recovery process. What floor in the hospital will I spend my recovery time on and how many patients on the same floor are having thoracic procedures?

68. How long will it take to recover?

Everyone will recover from surgery at their own pace, and recovery depends on a number of factors. Your overall medical condition prior to surgery will impact the time it takes to recover. Complications are a risk of any surgery, and if you experience any complications it may take you slightly longer to recover.

Exercising for about an hour a day is usually recommended. You may not be able to do that much at one time and may want to break it up into shorter segments with an aggregate of an hour a day. You may have to start with a shorter time and progressively increase to the recommended duration. Exercise is very important after surgery to prevent complications such as pneumonia and blood clots. Your doctor will advise you about walking in the hospital after surgery and continuing this at home after discharge. Moderate exercise can also help improve your appetite and fatigue following surgery.

If you are working and have taken time off from work for surgery, you may require 8 to 12 weeks prior to returning to your job. This will depend on the type of work you do on a day-to-day basis. Keep in mind, however, that it can be difficult to go back for "just a few hours" or a few days a week. Once there, you may be asked to do more than you are ready to do. Therefore, it is often better to take the maximum amount of time your doctor advises.

Bart's comment:

It took me approximately 2 months from the day I left the hospital until I went back to work. I work at a desk so there was not a great deal of manual labor involved in what I do.

69. What is laparoscopic surgery?

Laparoscopy is a type of surgery where small incisions are made into the abdominal wall and specially designed ports are placed through the incisions. A gas is then used to inflate the abdomen so that the organs and structures can be visualized with a telescope, and a camera is introduced into the abdominal cavity through a "port." Instruments are then placed through additional ports and, with the help of a camera, the abdominal cavity is visualized. Surgical procedures or biopsies can then be performed. Although healing of incisions takes a similar time period, the incisions are smaller and the pain/

discomfort may be less with laparoscopic surgery. In most cases, laparoscopy for diagnosis or small procedures is an outpatient procedure and patients go home the same day. They may experience some abdominal discomfort or shoulder pain, but these are minimal and usually subside after a day or two.

For patients with esophageal cancer, laparoscopy is most often performed as a diagnostic test to determine the extent of disease. In some patients, esophageal cancer can spread to the lymph nodes, abdominal wall, or liver, and for these patients an esophagectomy would not be the recommended treatment. A laparoscopy can determine if this spread has occurred and prevent unnecessary surgery. Research has found diagnostic laparoscopy to be a useful tool to detect if cancer has spread to the lymph nodes or other parts of the abdomen. Discuss with your surgeon if any of your staging tests (CAT, endoscopy, or PET scan) indicate that a diagnostic laparoscopy would be recommended.

Some surgeons are investigating utilizing a laparoscopic approach to perform an esophagectomy. This is a new procedure that requires specific skills from the surgeon, and the long-term results of these procedures are not known. Research is ongoing to determine if this approach is adequate for a cancer operation.

70. What is laser surgery or ablative therapy?

During **laser surgery** or ablative therapy, cancer is treated by procedures that destroy the cancerous tissue. Lasers or electrocoagulation are utilized to destroy the tissue. One instance where these procedures are used is for patients with Barrett's esophagus with dysplasia. This treatment

Laser surgery

A surgical procedure using a device that concentrates high energies into an intense narrow beam of nondivergent monochromatic electromagnetic radiation; used in microsurgery, cauterization, and diagnostic purposes.

has had mixed results. Ablation is successful in about half of the patients treated, but rates of recurrence at different centers differ widely. The difficulties of this type of treatment are related to the fact that this is a relatively new treatment and differences exist in ablation techniques. In addition, after treatment with ablation, the patient requires acid suppression therapy, either with surgery or with medications, to prevent the return of the Barrett's.

The benefits of this type of treatment are still being investigated, and until more is known, the treatment must still be considered experimental. If you have Barrett's esophagus with dysplasia, discuss with your gastroenterologist the benefits and risks of this type of treatment. As this is a new procedure and not all gastroenterologists or surgeons may be familiar with it, you may also want to find a center that has experience in this type of treatment for Barrett's esophagus.

71. Someone mentioned photodynamic therapy as a treatment for esophageal cancer. What is this?

Photodynamic therapy (PDT)

A type of surgery that uses an injection of photosensitizing drugs to highlight the cancerous cells and laser light through an endoscope to kill them.

Photosensitizing

A type of treatment where target cancer cells are illuminated by bioluminescent drugs.

Photodynamic therapy has been used as treatment for Barrett's esophagus with high-grade dysplasia or for palliation in advanced obstructing esophageal cancer. For this treatment, a type of laser light destroys cancer cells after the patient has been administered certain drugs that are **photosensitizing**. Treatment with photodynamic therapy is a two-step process. The first step involves intravenous injection of a photosensitizing agent. Photofrin (porfimer sodium) is a photosensitizing agent that is FDA approved in the United States for palliative treatment of advanced esophageal cancer. The agent remains in cancer cells for a longer period of time than it does in normal cells. The second step is to treat the area with cancer with a laser light. The laser light is directed to the area through an endoscope in a procedure similar to a regular endoscopy. When the cancer cells are exposed to laser light, the photosensitizing agent absorbs the light and the cancer cells are destroyed. Sometimes, a second endoscopy may be necessary to mechanically remove dead cells or debris. Timing of the light exposure is critical—it must be timed to occur when most of the photosensitizing agent has left the healthy cells but is still present in the cancer cells.

A side effect of the photosensitizing agent Photofrin is photosensitivity. The skin and eyes are sensitive to light for six weeks or more following injection of the drug. During this time, patients are at risk to develop damage to the skin or the eyes and must remain out of the sunlight and avoid bright indoor light. Patients are advised to wear dark sunglasses when outdoors or in bright light. Other temporary side effects can include coughing, difficulty swallowing, and abdominal pain.

The advantage of photodynamic therapy is that it causes minimal damage to normal tissue near the dysplasia or cancer. However, the laser light cannot penetrate deep into the tissues, and, therefore, this treatment is used to treat early superficial tumors or dysplasia, or to remove cancer cells that may be causing an obstruction in the esophagus.

72. How is photodynamic therapy used to treat high-grade dysplasia?

Photodynamic therapy (PDT) is the most common experimental treatment for patients with Barrett's esophagus and high-grade dysplasia. Dysplasia can be eliminated in more than 75% of patients treated with PDT. After treatment, patients need ongoing surveillance for persistent or recurrent Barrett's.

For patients with high-grade dysplasia, the risk of developing an invasive cancer is not inevitable but is high. Historically, patients with this condition faced two options: close endoscopic surveillance or surgical resection of the esophagus. Surgery is highly curative for high-grade dysplasia and early cancer, and for patients who can tolerate an esophagectomy, this is the preferred method of treatment. For patients who are not able to tolerate surgery, ablation therapy is an option. Recent research has found that this treatment holds promise for select patients with high-grade dysplasia who cannot tolerate surgery for medical reasons. As this is still considered an experimental treatment, long-term studies are needed to demonstrate whether this treatment will prevent esophageal cancer in these patients.

73. How is photodynamic therapy used to treat advanced esophageal cancer?

Cancer that has advanced within the esophagus can cause a blockage or obstruction that can lead to difficulty or inability to swallow, decreased oral intake, and aspiration of food or saliva into the lungs, which can lead to pneumonia. In some cases, palliative treatment can improve these symptoms and the patient's overall quality of life. Palliative treatment is meant to relieve symptoms and make the patient more comfortable, but is not meant as a cure for the disease.

Palliative treatment is meant to relieve symptoms and make the patient more comfortable, but is not meant as a cure for the disease.

One method of palliation that has been used for esophageal cancer is photodynamic therapy (PDT). When the tumor is within the esophagus and is causing obstruction or bleeding, PDT can be used to treat the tumor and remove some of the tissue, thus opening the obstruction or stopping the bleeding. The advantage of PDT over other treatments is that it can improve symptoms within days of treatment, there is minimal pain with the treatment, and PDT is administered in most cases on an outpatient basis. Disadvantages such as photosensitivity, risk of perforation of the esophagus, and the need for possible repeat treatments must be considered.

Other treatments for palliation of obstructing esophageal cancer include external beam radiation, laser therapy, or stents. Each has advantages and disadvantages, and a thorough discussion with your physician will help you decide which treatment is best for you (see Question 79 for more information on palliative treatment).

SIDE EFFECTS OF SURGICAL TREATMENT

74. I have trouble swallowing after surgery. What can I do?

After surgery, as the anastomosis (area where the esophagus was reconnected) heals, a stricture can form. A stricture is a narrowing or tightening of the esophagus. This can also occur after other treatments, including laser therapy or photodynamic therapy. After surgery, the anastomosis forms a scar. Consider the way the skin around a scar on your hand or knee pulls up or puckers. A similar process can occur in your esophagus, and as this area heals the tissue pulls and tightens. This can lead to difficulty swallowing.

One way to help prevent this from occurring is to eat solid foods. As you swallow solids, they will naturally help to stretch the esophagus and keep it open. A stricture can still develop even if you have been trying to eat solids. If you do start to experience difficulty swallowing, alert your surgeon or your nurse. They will assess what you are able to eat and when your difficulty occurs.

Treatment for a stricture can be done in your surgeon's office or as an outpatient procedure in the hospital. In some cases, your surgeon can see you in the office and, while you swallow, inserts a weighted tube, called a **bougie**, which will open the stricture. Sometimes several treatments are required to keep the esophagus open. For some patients who require repeated treatments, their surgeon will instruct them to repeat this procedure at home. In other cases, your surgeon may wish to stretch the esophagus during an endoscopy at the hospital. This is similar to a regular endoscopy, and a balloon is used to open the esophagus. Your surgeon will discuss which procedure is best for your situation.

Bart's comment:

If you are experiencing problems with swallowing, where food seems to be taking a long time to clear your esophagus, it could be that scar tissue that formed where your surgery took place could be tightening, so you will need a dilation to stretch your opening. This is a procedure that can be done either in your surgeon's office or in the hospital. During the first year of my recovery I had a dilation done four times, three times in the hospital and one time in my surgeon's office.

75. What are some other side effects of surgery?

Esophageal surgery has other potential side effects. Some are temporary and some will require permanent lifestyle changes. Your surgeon will discuss with you possible side

Bougie

A cylindrical instrument used for dilating constricted areas in tubular organs (such as the esophagus).

effects and the risks of each, given your situation and planned treatment.

Some patients experience a change in their voices following surgery. Some changes in your voice may be temporary; however, some may be lasting. The location of your tumor will determine whether your voice is affected by surgery. If your tumor is located at the top of your esophagus, your surgeon will discuss the implications of surgery on your voice.

It is not unusual for someone who has received anesthesia to experience a decrease or loss of appetite. Those who have had esophagectomies may take longer to regain their appetites. Also, because the gastrointestinal tract has been reconfigured and the stomach is smaller, patients often complain of feelings of fullness and discomfort when ingesting much smaller portions. These symptoms do resolve with time. It is recommended that people who have esophagectomies eat six small meals a day (see Question 81 for more specifics on diet changes after an esophagectomy).

Patients who have had their esophagus removed will need to adjust their sleep position. In most cases, when the esophagus is removed as part of an esophagectomy, the sphincter, or valve, at the lower end of the esophagus is removed as well. Normally this valve prevents acid and stomach contents from coming back up into the esophagus and lungs. Without this valve there is a possibility that if you sleep flat, some stomach acid or contents could travel up the esophagus and leak into the lungs. This leaking can lead to serious complications such as pneumonia. In order to prevent this, it is recommended that you sleep with the head of your bed elevated about

Patients who have had their esophagus removed will need to adjust their sleep position.

10 to 12 inches. This change is permanent and will need to be maintained for the rest of your life.

Raising your bed to this height requires more than just extra pillows. There are several methods to raise the head of your bed. One is to place blocks or risers under the two posts at the head of the bed. An advantage of this is that the entire bed is then on an incline and you won't be able to "wiggle down" to a flat position. You can also purchase a wedge that will raise the top part of your body. It is important to consider a wedge that raises your entire torso, from your hips to your head. Wedges are available that only raise the head and shoulders, but this would not be adequate for people who have had their esophagus removed. Some wedges are even inflatable and can be packed in your suitcase for travel. A good company to check for a wedge is Back Be Nimble (*http://www.backbenimble.com* or 800-639-3746). You can also check your local medical supply pharmacy for wedges.

Bart's comment:

My experience after my adenocarcinoma surgery has been that the only time I find my voice changing is after I eat, especially when I have eaten too much. Your stomach, which now starts in the middle of your chest, fights for space with your lungs, and not getting enough air into your lungs can impact your projection of words.

After my surgery, which took a portion of my stomach as well as the cancer in my esophagus, I found that I had to eat smaller meals and eat more often to get the nourishment my body needed while still paying attention to the new size of my stomach. A well-balanced meal is always important, and more so with a limited amount of food you can take in at a given point of time. Drinking, which also is important, should be kept to a minimum during your eating, only sipping a drink during this time. The major part of your fluid intake should occur two hours before and two hours after your meals.

Also, you should finish your food intake for the day at least two hours before you go to bed. In this way you give your system time to digest the food, so it does not sit in your stomach overnight, which could cause acid or bile reflux to occur.

If your surgery involved taking a portion of your stomach, then the valve that holds your food down undoubtedly had to be removed. Since there is no replacement for that valve, you need to sleep at a 30° incline so the food in your stomach stays there. This position can be accomplished in several ways. You can buy and sleep on a wedge. You can put wood blocks under the head portion of the bed that will in effect raise the head portion of the bed so that the entire bed is at a 30° angle. The other option would be to purchase adjustable beds so you can set your bed at one level and your partner can set their section of the bed at the level they desire.

76. What is "dumping"?

Dumping syndrome is a common occurrence following surgery and is also called rapid gastric emptying. This occurs when the lower end of the small intestine fills too quickly with undigested food. Dumping can occur either "early" or "late." Early dumping occurs soon after a meal and symptoms include nausea, vomiting, bloating, and diarrhea. Late dumping occurs one to three hours after eating and symptoms include weakness, sweating, and dizziness. Although both types are possible after surgery, late dumping is more common.

Bart's comment:

I found that eating too many carbohydrates at one time has caused my dumping. As I understand it, your stomach passes

Dumping syndrome

Post-surgical rapid gastric emptying; early dumping symptoms include nausea, vomiting, bloating, and diarrhea; late dumping symptoms include weakness, sweating, and dizziness.

the food quickly and at that time insulin is being pumped into your stomach, and there is no food for it to interact with, which causes the dumping. I can feel it coming on, as I will begin to sweat and feel light-headed. I will drink orange juice and eat some protein like peanuts or peanut butter cookies, and within 20 minutes the dumping feeling is gone.

77. What should the postoperative patient do to minimize the discomfort associated with dumping syndrome?

If you do experience dumping, changing your eating habits may help. Try eating more slowly or eating smaller, more frequent meals. Also, avoiding high fat or high sugar foods can help. In some cases your doctor can prescribe medications to slow your digestion. It is a good idea to keep some juice and a snack, such as nuts, available with you at all times in case you start to feel symptoms of weakness or dizziness. If you do experience these symptoms, discuss them with your doctor.

There are several dietary changes that you can try if you experience dumping that may help to minimize it or prevent it from occurring. Limiting fluids with your meals to ½ cup may help. Some people have found relief by avoiding lactose in the first months after surgery. Also, avoiding temperature extremes in food and increasing soluble fiber may help prevent dumping syndrome from occurring.

Bart's comment:

Dumping is a product of your eating habits. If you eat too much sugar or carbohydrates and you eat too fast, you do not give your system proper time to digest what you have eaten.

As a result, your stomach just releases what you have eaten into your lower intestines and a dumping syndrome ensues.

You know that you are experiencing a dumping syndrome when you feel weak, have shortness of breath, are sweating profusely, and need to rest from the overall weak feeling. Usually some orange juice or a small candy or anything sweet will get you out of this feeling within 20 or 30 minutes.

78. What is palliative treatment?

Palliative treatment is given not with the intent to cure, but with the intent to prolong survival, shrink the tumor, and improve symptoms. Generally, chemotherapy for advanced esophageal cancer is palliative treatment. It is administered with the intent to shrink the tumor or at least keep it stable. In doing so, one hopes to prolong life and decrease symptoms, thereby improving quality of life.

79. What palliative treatments are used to treat cancer of the esophagus?

Unfortunately, many people with cancer of the esophagus are diagnosed after the cancer has spread from the esophagus and are not candidates for curative treatment. For these individuals, the goal of treatment is relief of symptoms to improve quality of life. Chemotherapy, surgery, and radiation can all be used as palliative treatments. The choice of treatment is based on each technique's advantages and disadvantages, the area to be treated, as well as the patient's overall condition. Your doctor will individualize treatment to your specific case. Discuss with him or her the plan for treatment as well as the advantages and disadvantages.

Your doctor will individualize treatment to your specific case.

125

Surgery

Surgery is a difficult decision when cancer is at an advanced stage. Occasionally, a palliative esophagectomy or surgery to bypass the esophagus may be considered. The goal of surgery in this situation is the relief of dysphagia. Some studies have found that over 80% of patients had complete and lasting relief of dysphagia following palliative esophagectomy. Despite these benefits, surgery carries a high risk of morbidity and mortality in these patients and requires careful consideration.

Radiation Therapy

Radiation therapy is an important method of palliation for patients with esophageal cancer. In 50% to 70% of patients, radiation can lead to relief of dysphagia. An important factor to consider is that it takes about four to six weeks for the effects of radiation therapy to be seen. Thus, this would not be an appropriate treatment for someone with a complete obstruction who requires immediate relief. Complications of radiation therapy are esophagitis, narrowing of the esophagus, and fistula. Radiation therapy is noninvasive. This is advantageous to patients; however, it does require time and travel to the hospital every day for several weeks.

Brachytherapy

Brachytherapy is a type of radiation therapy where radiation is delivered directly to the tumor by radioactive seeds that are placed directly in or near the tumor. Brachytherapy can directly treat an esophageal tumor and shortens treatment time. The radioactive seeds can be permanent when they are implanted directly into the tumor or they can be placed in a hollow tube and passed near the tumor for a set number of minutes. A complication of brachytherapy is esophagitis. The majority of patients treated with brachytherapy will have relief of their dysphagia.

Brachytherapy may be combined with external beam radiation therapy. The goal of this treatment is to improve the local control of the tumor. This combination can restore normal swallowing in the majority of patients.

Chemoradiation

Chemotherapy has been utilized alone or in combination with radiation therapy in the palliative treatment of esophageal cancer. Research has found that this approach provides good, long-lasting relief of dysphagia. Toxicity from **chemoradiation** is a concern and is higher when the treatments are combined than when they are given as single treatments.

Dilatation

Dilatation, or stretching of the esophagus, is an important first step in the palliative treatment of patients with obstructing esophageal tumors. This treatment can offer relief of dysphagia with a low risk of complications. The duration of relief is short, so dilatation is rarely used alone as a palliative treatment. The advantages of this treatment are its simplicity, availability, low cost, ability to be performed in the outpatient setting, and applicability to many types of tumors.

Stents

Plastic or metal stents are often utilized for palliative treatment. These can be a thread, rod, or catheter that is inserted into the wall of the esophagus to keep it open when it becomes constricted (see **Figure 8**). Advantages of this treatment are its simplicity, short hospitalization, and immediate improvement in swallowing. Complications rarely occur but include perforation, hemorrhage, pneumonia, and tube dislocation. A disadvantage of this treatment is that the tumor can overgrow the stent and that food may become impacted. Recently, metal stents

Chemoradiation
Chemotherapy used in combination with radiation therapy.

Dilatation
(also dilation) An outpatient treatment used to stretch the esophagus.

TREATMENT OPTIONS

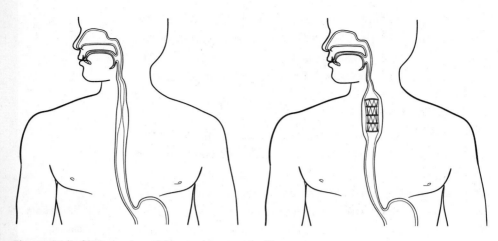

Figure 8 (Left) Narrowing of the esophagus caused by tumor.
(Right) Esophageal stent placement.

that reduce some of the complications seen with plastic prostheses have been introduced.

Laser Therapy

Lasers are used to destroy the tumor and open the esophagus to allow for better swallowing. Traditionally, a type of laser called the Nd:YAG laser was utilized. This laser is placed at or near the tumor to destroy the cancer cells. The advantage of laser therapy is its high success rate with low complications. Relief is almost immediate and the treatment can be repeated indefinitely. Laser therapy is performed as an outpatient procedure with local anesthesia. Complications are rare but include perforation, bleeding, and fistula formation.

Photodynamic Therapy

Photodynamic therapy is also used in palliative treatment of esophageal cancer (see Question 71).

Each palliative treatment has advantages and disadvantages and may be indicated for specific symptoms. Your physician will discuss with you the techniques he or she is recommending and why.

80. Am I at risk for a blood clot? What is a pulmonary embolism?

A blood clot that occurs in a deep-lying vein in the leg or pelvis is known as a **deep vein thrombosis** (DVT). If the blood clot breaks off and travels up through the heart and into the lungs, it is called a **pulmonary embolism (PE)**. A pulmonary embolism is a potentially serious condition because if it is a large blood clot, it can block off a blood vessel going to the lung and cause significant problems with breathing, or even death.

Lots of things can cause a DVT, particularly in the elderly, including poor circulation, sitting for long periods of time, or being bedridden following surgery. For unclear reasons, patients with cancer have a higher tendency to get blood clots. If you have had a blood clot, your doctor can prescribe an anticoagulant to treat it.

Bart's comment:

I developed a blood clot several years after my esophagectomy that covered my entire left leg. Blood thinners were used as the method to treat blood clots. A filter was inserted so that if the blood clot were to travel, the filter would prevent it from getting to a vital organ. I was on these thinners for a year and then we decided to stop these thinners.

Deep vein thrombosis

A blood clot that occurs in a deep-lying vein in the leg or pelvis.

Pulmonary embolism (PE)

A blood clot that has broken away from the blood vessel wall and travels into the lung; a large clot can cause breathing problems and even death.

TREATMENT OPTIONS

PART SIX

Living with Esophageal Cancer

I don't seem to have much of an appetite after treatment. How can I improve my appetite and nutrition during and after treatment?

Will I be able to work during and after treatment?

How do I get my life back to normal?

How can I cope psychologically with cancer? I feel depressed. Is this common?

More . . .

81. I don't seem to have much of an appetite after treatment. How can I improve my appetite and nutrition during and after treatment?

Treatment for esophageal cancer can affect your appetite in different ways. Chemotherapy can cause nausea or may alter your taste for food. Radiation can cause irritation to your esophagus and make swallowing painful. An esophagectomy reduces the size of your stomach and may change the rate at which food leaves your stomach and is absorbed by the body. In addition, each of these treatments can lead to a decrease in your general appetite, and you may not feel you have a taste for food. In fact, some patients have even said they developed an aversion to food following treatment.

Maintaining your nutritional level and weight during and after treatment is a challenge, and is vitally important to recovery and healing.

Maintaining your nutritional level and weight during and after treatment is a challenge, and is vitally important to recovery and healing. We will provide some general tips to increase your appetite and maintain your nutrition, and then give some specific advice of each type of treatment.

If you have difficulty swallowing or pain when swallowing, discuss these symptoms with your doctor. Some of the following tips may be difficult to try if you are having trouble swallowing. In that case, it may be helpful to meet with a dietitian or nutritionist who works with your medical team. He or she can be a valuable resource as you navigate treatment and recovery.

Maintaining Calories and Stimulating Appetite

- Large meals can seem overwhelming, so try frequent, small meals instead of three large meals.
- Drink beverages high in calories such as milkshakes, fruit juices, and nectars instead of diet drinks, coffee, or tea.
- Keep snack foods that you like readily available at home and work.
- Eat your favorite foods any time of the day—if you feel like an omelet for dinner, have one.
- Pleasant aromas such as bread baking or bacon frying can help to stimulate your appetite.
- Avoid foods that are labeled "low fat," "nonfat," or "diet."
- Snack on dried fruits and nuts or add them to hot cereals, ice cream, or salads.
- Add sour cream, half-and-half, or heavy cream to mashed potatoes, cake and cookie recipes, pancake batter, sauces, gravies, soups, and casseroles.

Increasing Protein in Your Diet

Protein can help your body to heal from surgery or wounds and helps your body to function efficiently.

- Eat foods high in protein such as chicken, fish, pork, beef, eggs, milk, cheese, beans, and tofu.
- Drink "double milk" by adding 1 envelope of non-fat dry milk powder to 1 quart of milk and blending. Refrigerate after blending.
- Add powdered milk to cream soups, mashed potatoes, milkshakes, and casseroles.

- Snack on cheese or nut butters (such as peanut butter, cashew butter, etc.) with crackers, apples, bananas, raisins, or celery.
- Add chickpeas, kidney beans, tofu, hard-cooked eggs, nuts, cooked meats, or fish to your salads.
- Add grated cheese to sauces, vegetables, soups, baked or mashed potatoes, casseroles, and salads.
- Add wheat germ to cereals, casseroles, and yogurt.

Bart's comment:

I found that exercising increased my appetite post-surgery. In fact exercising can be the solution for a lot of experiences post-surgery. I found by exercising I healed quicker and my appetite came back quicker, and the overall feeling of depression was experienced fewer times.

82. How will chemotherapy and radiation affect my nutrition and digestive system? Can these side effects be managed?

Chemotherapy

Many chemotherapy agents can affect the digestive system and cause nausea and vomiting, diarrhea, sore mouth, dry mouth, weight loss, and changes in the taste of food. These side effects depend on the drugs you receive and doses used and vary from person to person. New medications are available to manage some of these symptoms. Some patients may experience very mild symptoms or no symptoms at all. The tips that follow can help to manage some of these side effects, but if you do experience any of these, discuss them with your nurse and your doctor (see Question 54 for more side effects of chemotherapy).

Bart's comment:

The chemotherapy protocol is what I like to call "patient friendly." They usually are given once a week so people can continue to work during their treatments. Patients can work the remaining part of the week, and my experience in talking to some patients has been that they can work even on the day they take their treatment. This is a good area to measure the progress that has been made over the last few years.

My chemotherapy protocol was 24 hours a day for 5 days a week, for 6 straight weeks. While I was going through this protocol I was also taking radiation therapy each day (28 treatments) as well.

I had very little side effects from my chemotherapy treatment. At one point in the protocol, I asked my doctors if we were sure that the treatment was working and they assured me that it was, and in fact my tumor reduced in size as a result of the therapy that I was given.

Radiation Therapy

Radiation to the esophagus can cause a sore mouth, sore throat, difficulty swallowing, and taste changes. Follow the tips below to help manage these side effects. In addition to the tips listed, it would be helpful to avoid acidic foods such as orange juice and tomatoes, which may irritate the esophagus (see Question 59 for more side effects of radiation).

Bart's comment:

I did not have any bad side effects from my radiation therapy. It was painless for me. I did not have any radiation burns and, along with the chemotherapy I took, overall it reduced the size of my tumor from 5 cm to 1 cm.

Nutrition Tips to Manage Side Effects During Chemotherapy and Radiation

- Diarrhea: If you experience diarrhea, check with your doctor before treating it yourself. Drink at least 8 cups (8 oz. each) of liquid to replace water and electrolytes you may be losing. Try well-cooked, pureed, and peeled canned vegetables and fruits such as bananas, peeled apples, and diluted juices. Try white breads, cereals, rice, pasta, and farina. Avoid whole grain breads, breads with nuts or seeds, and fatty breads or pastries. Avoid large amounts of sugar, spices, rich gravies, and caffeine.

- Sore or dry mouth: Mouth dryness or sores can make eating difficult or painful. For a dry mouth, try soft and pureed foods and cold foods. Sugar-free mints or gum can help to stimulate saliva production for a dry mouth. For mouth sores, try bland, soft, pureed foods such as creamed soups, casseroles, macaroni and cheese, and scrambled eggs. For both a dry mouth and mouth sores, avoid rough or dry foods such as meat without sauce, crackers, pretzels, and raw fruits and vegetables.

- Taste changes: Changes in taste vary from person to person, but the most common changes are bitter and metallic tastes in the mouth. Occasionally, food may seem to have no taste at all. When food seems tasteless, use spices and flavoring, as tolerated. For example, add sauces and condiments, such as soy sauce and Creole spice. Marinate meats in salad dressing or another favorite sauce. Try herbs such as rosemary, basil, and oregano, mint, and different types of mustard. Try sour and tart foods as these may help to stimulate taste. Look for recipes from different regional American and international cuisines in the grocery store and on the Internet. If you have a bitter or metallic taste in the mouth, rinse with water before meals. If meats taste bitter, try marinating them in fruit-based sauces or fruit juices. Use plastic utensils to reduce a metallic taste, and try sugar-free mints or gum.

- Nausea: Nausea is a common side effect of treatment, and medications are available to help control nausea. Talk with your doctor or nurse if you have nausea before trying the following suggestions. Try high-carbohydrate, low-fat, bland foods such as gelatin, dry toast, skinless chicken, light pasta salads, and popsicles. Avoid high-fat, spicy, or overly sweet foods and fatty meats and fried foods.

83. How will surgery affect my digestive system? How can I manage these side effects?

Surgery results in two physical changes that impact the way you eat and digest food. The first is that your stomach will be smaller, which will lead to feeling full more quickly after eating than you did before surgery. Second, the valve that controls the rate at which food leaves your stomach and enters your intestines may be altered, which means nutrients may not be absorbed as well as before. Before or after your surgery, you should meet with a dietitian to discuss your particular needs. Some general tips follow.

Before or after your surgery, you should meet with a dietitian to discuss your particular needs.

- Eat six or seven small meals daily instead of three main meals. This will help you to eat the proper amount of food even though your stomach is smaller. The amount of food you are able to eat at each meal will increase over time but may not reach your pre-surgery capacity.

- Eat slowly and chew your food thoroughly. This helps digestion and lets you know when you are full, so you can stop eating before you feel uncomfortable.
- Drink no more than 4 ounces of liquid at meal times. This allows you to eat more solid foods and slows the passage of food to the small intestine.
- Drink liquids before and after meals to prevent dehydration. You should drink about 8 to 10 cups of fluid a day.
- Eat sweets in moderation. Sugar in drinks and foods such as sodas, fruit juices, candy, and cake can cause food to flow more quickly into the small intestine, which can lead to cramping, stomach pain, or diarrhea (see Question 60 for more information on this side effect).
- Test your tolerance for fats. Try a small amount first and increase slowly. You may have trouble digesting large amounts of fat.
- Sometimes people become lactose-intolerant after surgery. This usually goes away after a few months. After surgery, gradually introduce dairy products into your diet. If you think you may be lactose intolerant, contact a dietitian for guidance.

After surgery and when you are able to tolerate liquids, you may want to start with soft, tender foods. As the esophagus heals, the area that was reconnected (anastomosis) will form a scar and may shrink or tighten. Eating solid foods will help to keep this open. If you experience coughing or the sensation of food getting stuck when you swallow, inform your doctor.

During an esophagectomy, the valve between your stomach and esophagus (the gastroesophageal sphincter) is removed. This can cause contents of your stomach to move upwards and enter the esophagus. It is important to prevent this. Sit upright during and for at least 30 minutes after meals. Wear loose fitting clothing and allow at least two hours between your last meal and bedtime. Keep the head of your bed elevated to a 30° angle.

Bart's comment:

This is major surgery and I was in the hospital for 10 days. The key element to being in the hospital is you need to work while you are there. Walking, coughing, and using the breathing machine are all things I had to do to avoid complications in the recovery process.

When you first go home after surgery, you will find that you will need to eat more meals, and you will need to eat by the clock since you will not have an appetite. If the clock says 12 noon, have half of a sandwich; at 2:00, have the other half. In effect you are eating each meal—breakfast, lunch, and dinner—in two sittings. As your time from surgery lengthens, you will begin to get your appetite back. I have found for myself that exercising during the recovery process will bring my appetite back sooner.

84. When can I consider myself cured of esophageal cancer?

Surviving cancer is a process and it is difficult to pinpoint a time when you can consider yourself "cured." As you transition from treatment to life after treatment, you may face many challenges. More and more hospitals and community agencies are focusing on support services and educational programs for individuals who have completed their treatment for cancer. Contact your hospital or local American Cancer Society for local resources. Good Web sites for survivorship information are the National Coalition for Cancer Survivorship (*http://www.canceradvocacy.org*) and the National Cancer Institute's Office of Cancer Survivorship (*http://cancercontrol.cancer.gov/ocs*) and the Lance Armstrong Foundation (*http://www.livestrong.org*).

Bart's comment:

I do not consider myself as being cured of esophageal cancer, but rather, I consider myself as having successfully gone through chemotherapy, radiation, and surgery. All tests taken from surgery to date (CAT scans and endoscopies) have indicated that no further cancer has been identified in my body.

In the first year, I took a CAT scan every six months with an alternating endoscope every six months as well, in effect visiting my surgeon four times that first year. I repeated these tests on a six-month basis. This is to say, I visited my surgeon twice the second and third years. We continued this through my fourth year of recovery. I am now eight years out from surgery, and my surgeon has indicated I should have a CAT scan every 2 years.

85. Will I be able to work during and after treatment?

Surgery usually requires a 10- to 14-day hospital stay and a 6- to 8-week recovery before going back to work.

How individuals respond to treatment varies greatly. Chemotherapy may be given from one to several days a week. Most often it is given on an outpatient basis, but occasionally patients are required to stay overnight in the hospital. Some patients are able to work throughout chemotherapy and take only a few days off, while others need more time. Radiation therapy is given Monday through Friday, and even though the treatment may only take a few minutes, the distance to the facility must be considered. Surgery usually requires a 10- to 14-day hospital stay and a 6- to 8-week recovery before going back to work. Your doctor will outline your treatment schedule, which will allow you to estimate if you'll need time away from work.

If you believe that you may need some time away from work during your treatment and recovery, you may need to talk with your supervisor about taking sick leave or perhaps changing your responsibilities during this time. If you are unable to work full-time and must switch to part-time hours, speak to your company's human resources or benefits department staff. Be aware that the Family and Medical Leave Act allows eligible employees up to a total of 12 weeks of unpaid leave during any 12-month period. For information about this legislation, contact the human resources department where you work or the United States Department of Labor (*http://www.dol.gov/dol/topic/benefits-leave/fmla.htm*).

You may be concerned about discussing your diagnosis with your supervisor or coworkers. The Americans with Disabilities Act protects you from discrimination at work and requires that employers make reasonable adjustments as long as you can perform the essential functions of the job. Unfortunately, some employers do not always respond in the way we hope they will or in the way the law requires. If you do need to talk with a supervisor or coworker, prepare ahead for the conversation. First, determine how you can get the most important parts of your job done. Then, determine how you need to alter the hours you work to balance getting the job done with taking care of your medical needs. Being open at the beginning can be helpful in obtaining information about your rights and benefits. If you are not comfortable talking about this with your supervisor, talk with someone in the human resources department. If conflicts arise, you may need to contact an attorney for assistance. For more information about the Americans with Disabilities Act and how it applies to you, contact the United States Department of Justice (*http://www.ada.gov* or 1-800-514-0301) or the United States Equal Employment Opportunity Commission (*http://www.eeoc.gov* or 1-800-669-4000).

Bart's comment:

Most people can work during the chemotherapy and radiation treatments they encounter. After surgery, you may need 2 to 3 months to get back into a working mode. Some patients have done this sooner, and to a great extent it is up to how the patient feels and what he thinks he can handle. For me I was released from the hospital on May 27th and went back to work on August 1st.

86. How do I get my life back to normal?

The transition from treatment to normal life can include many conflicting emotions. If your treatment has been successful, you probably will be relieved and happy. At the same time, you may feel distressed and this emotional conflict is not unusual. You probably have made friendships with those involved in your care as well as other patients and their families. Now that you are not going to your healthcare facility regularly, you may not see them as often or perhaps ever see them again. What had become a routine focus of your life is changing. This is a time of transition. It is normal to find it difficult to finish treatment and carry on with your life.

A support group may be helpful to you at this time. Here, you may find other cancer survivors who are facing similar circumstances. You will also be able to reach out to newly diagnosed patients. This effort to help others can make you feel good about yourself and remind you about how far you have come. If your anxiety causes you to feel depressed or interferes with your functioning, you should talk to your doctor and ask whether counseling or medication might help to alleviate your distress. You should also let your family and friends know that you still need their support even though you are no longer in treatment. They may assume everything is okay unless you take the time to explain your ongoing needs.

An important part of getting your life back to normal is to be vigilant about your follow-up care and "wellness care." Although follow-up care for cancer of the esophagus varies among doctors, you should be aware of your doctor's recommendations for office visits, scans, and follow-up tests. In addition to your cancer concerns, you should discuss "wellness care" with your doctor. It is important that you take good care of your general health so that you can be strong in your survival.

What will be most effective for getting back to normal and resolving your emotional distress is the passage of time. As each day passes, you will feel more comfortable with your status as a cancer survivor. You will adjust to the emotional, physical, and social changes brought about by your cancer experience and find a new equilibrium—a new normal—that will carry you through your life.

Bart's comment:
I like to say that my life has a slightly different definition of normal. I can now eat the same foods I ate before, and I can play golf as I did before, although I am probably three strokes worse. So why do I say a "slightly different" definition of normal? Simply put, I now eat more than the three meals a day because my stomach is smaller than it was before surgery. Immediately after surgery, I was eating 6 meals a

day, which now after 4 years post-surgery has been reduced to three meals a day with a snack or two in between because my stomach has stretched since surgery.

Another slightly different routine than what I had before is with sleeping. I now sleep on an angle of approximately 30 degrees. My wife and I have adjustable beds. When we sleep we keep them at different angles but when they are placed flat they will give the appearance of being a king size bed.

When you think about these two changes, eating smaller meals and sleeping on an angle, they are changes for the better that people who have not gone through this treatment should also follow. Eating smaller meals is good for everyone, and sleeping with a small elevation is also good for everyone.

87. Will I be able to do the things I used to do, such as travel, go out to eat, and play sports?

You will be able to do as much of any activity you would like after being diagnosed with cancer of the esophagus. You may need to modify your activities during treatment, depending on how you feel.

Immediately after treatment, it is best to check with your doctor before traveling long distances. After being cleared, you're free to travel where you would like! As always, it is best to verify with your insurance company the policy for health-related emergencies while away from home and to know the location of the closest medical facility. If you've had an esophagectomy you will need to keep the head of your bed elevated. Extra pillows may not be enough; some medical supply companies sell inflatable wedges that pack easily for travel. Check with your local medical supply retailer or try Back Be Nimble (see the Appendix) for an inflatable wedge that is convenient for traveling.

Eating out is a good way to relax and see friends and family. If you have difficulty swallowing, order softer foods or ask for sauces or gravies on your entrée. If you are only able to eat small meals, order an appetizer and salad or share a dinner with a family member or friend. Leftovers are a great snack for later!

As we've talked about in other questions, exercise is a great way to build and maintain your strength during and after treatment. Certainly pace yourself, and start slow if you haven't exercised in a while or if you are just starting to exercise after not feeling well. It is always a good idea to have a companion with you in case you need anything. If you have any questions about when to start exercising following treatment, discuss them with your doctor.

Bart's comment:

The answer to all these questions is yes. You can travel, but keep in mind that you need to sleep on an angle, so you need to tell the hotel that you need additional pillows. You can also purchase a portable wedge. These wedges come with a pump and they are easy to blow-up. When you are finished using them, they will deflate and fit in a small compartment of your suitcase.

Going out to eat is also doable. Here you need to remember that a full course meal of appetizer, soup or salad, main entrée, and dessert is something you more than likely cannot do, but if you pace yourself and do not eat everything at each course, you could certainly enjoy all the courses.

I retired as of the end of 2007 so I am able to play golf twice a week. I find my game has not improved with this increase of play, and I still attribute my poor play to this cancer, but that is not really the case!

88. Will I continue to have acid reflux following treatment?

You may continue to have reflux, but this depends on the type of treatment you received and your general medical condition. If you've had surgery, the reflux is not usually caused by stomach acid but by bile.

Bile reflux occurs when bile, a digestive fluid produced in the liver, flows upward from your small intestine into your stomach and esophagus, where it can cause inflammation. The signs and symptoms of bile reflux are similar to those of acid reflux and include sour taste in mouth, nausea, and vomiting bile. It cannot be completely controlled by changes in diet or lifestyle. Your surgeon can prescribe medications to help prevent this and alleviate any symptoms you may have. If you do experience reflux during or after treatment, discuss it with your doctor.

Bart's comment:

Because the surgery removes several acid-producing glands, the likelihood of getting acid reflux is remote. However, bile reflux is a possibility and if that persists, you need to see your doctor, as there are medications that can be taken to protect your esophagus from the effects of bile reflux. I have experienced this bile reflux and it is similar to the acid reflux you may have experienced. It has occurred at night for me, and I found that if I ate very late and went to bed less then 2 hours after eating I would experience this bile reflux. Once I realized this, I make sure that I have a 2 hour gap between the time I stop eating and the time I go to bed.

89. *How can I cope psychologically with cancer? I feel depressed. Is this common?*

Just as each individual is different, each person's response to the diagnosis of cancer is different. It is normal to feel scared, depressed, angry, or any number of other emotions after being diagnosed with cancer. Developing a coping strategy can help you through difficult times during treatment and recovery. Relaxation techniques, such as meditation, can be useful while waiting for treatments to begin or to see your doctor in the office. Communicating openly and honestly with your friends and family can help you to gain strength from each other. Some people may prefer to discuss emotions and feelings with someone other than a close friend or family member. Professionals, such as social workers or psychologists, are good resources to discuss your feelings and can help you to develop effective coping strategies that work for you. A source of spiritual support can also be a valuable resource for difficult times. In addition, set aside some time to be alone as well as time to do activities you enjoy. Don't let cancer control your life—try to live as normally as possible and appreciate the good things in your life. If you do find you are having difficulty coping or are feeling depressed, discuss it with your doctor so that you can be referred to the appropriate person for assistance.

It is normal to feel scared, depressed, angry, or any number of other emotions after being diagnosed with cancer.

Bart's comment:

Depression has a way of finding its way into a cancer patient's thought process. No matter how much control you think you have, when cancer strikes it renders you helpless, and as such you can become depressed because you seemingly lose control. I have found an aggressive regimen of exercise can fight off the depression feelings you can develop. Being around a supportive group of family and friends also helps in handling the depression that may occur. There are social workers attached to your local cancer centers who are trained to recognize depression and plan an appropriate course of action, and if depression persists you should avail yourself of these services.

I also developed during my cancer treatment certain songs that I would like to hear that would give me the strength to fight depression. I also would watch a film called "Rudy" and this got me out of the "poor me" state that occasionally I found myself in.

90. Are support groups available?

Support groups are a good way for patients and families to face the challenges and uncertainties that are common following a cancer diagnosis. Support groups can help you feel less alone and can help you cope with diagnosis, treatment, and recovery. There are many support services offered by hospitals, cancer centers, community agencies, and private groups. Some groups are general cancer support groups while others are more specialized, such as a group for men with cancer, or may be specific to a certain type of cancer. Because cancer of the esophagus is a more rare type of cancer, it may be difficult to find a group specific to the patient with esophageal cancer. Contact the closest cancer center to you or your local American Cancer Society for a list of local support groups.

Support groups are often led by professionals, such as social workers, nurses, or psychologists, but they can also be led by patients and survivors. Some groups are strictly supportive, where participants discuss their feelings, reactions, and how they are coping. Other groups have an educational component and may address symptom management or educational needs of the participants. Groups vary in size, approach, and how often they meet. Many of these support groups are free but some do require a fee. Check with your insurance company to find out if your plan will cover the cost. It is important for you to find a group that is comfortable and convenient for you and that meets your needs. More support groups are being offered online and over the telephone to accommodate all patients. CancerCare is an organization that offers professional counseling individually or through professionally facilitated support groups. Both of these services are available online, through the telephone, and on-site in New York, Long Island, New Jersey, and Connecticut. All CancerCare services are free of charge. You can find more information at *http://www.cancercare.org* or 800-813-HOPE.

Bart's comment:

There are organizations and Web sites that you can utilize that will keep you in touch with other esophageal cancer patients. There is nothing like talking to a patient who is several years out from surgery to see how they coped with a problem that you are currently experiencing.

91. What support is available for my significant other and family?

Family and friends are also affected when someone they care about is diagnosed with cancer. Just as their loved one may benefit from support, they may also benefit from talking with a professional or with other families who are having similar experiences. Some support groups are designed specifically for families and friends of people diagnosed with cancer. Others may encourage family members and patients to participate in the same group. In addition to your local hospital or American Cancer Society, the National Cancer Institute has a fact sheet about services for people with cancer that lists organizations that provide different support groups. The NCI fact sheet entitled "National Organizations that Offer Services to People with Cancer and Their Families" is available on the Internet (*http://cis.nci.nih.gov/fact/ 8_1.htm*) or by calling the Cancer Information Service (1-800-4-CANCER). The National Family Caregivers Association (*http://www.nfcacares.org*, 800-896-3650) supports family caregivers by providing education and information, support and validation, public awareness, and advocacy.

Bart's comment:

There are several support groups that cater to patients and their families when it comes to esophageal cancer. Memorial Sloan-Kettering has a post-treatment support group available every couple of months. In addition, there are patient-oriented support groups where patients can become part of an e-mail network and share their experiences and questions with fellow patients. You can check their Web sites at http://www.eccafe.org *and* http://www.fightec.org.

92. What medical insurance issues am I likely to face?

Medical insurance can be complicated, and navigating your insurance coverage and policies can be overwhelming at times. With any serious illness, it is important to review your coverage because there may be restrictions as to which doctors and facilities are covered by your plan. If you have insurance through your employer, it may be helpful to contact your benefits department and ask a representative to help you understand your coverage. They may be able to advocate for you directly with the insurance company and could help with any difficulties you experience. Some questions you may want to ask your insurance company are:

- Can I see any doctor or go to any hospital, or only those in your plan?
- How much more will I have to pay if I would like to use a doctor outside your plan ("out of network")?
- Do I have coverage for a second opinion?
- Do I need authorization before having diagnostic tests or treatments? If so, what is the process for doing this?
- What coverage do I have for prescription medications?

Your hospital may have a financial counselor who can help to determine the estimated costs of your care. You may be able to work with them to calculate what you will have to pay out-of-pocket based on your insurance coverage. If you are not able to pay this fee, discuss how you can work out a realistic payment plan. If you have difficulty paying for care, meet with a social worker to find out what financial assistance is available. You may be entitled to government or charitable assistance, and the American Cancer Society or Cancer Care may also be able to provide assistance.

The cost of prescription medications can be significant, and many pharmaceutical companies have assistance programs to provide medication at a reduced cost. To find out about financial assistance available for a particular medication, ask your nurse or social worker for information. The American Cancer Society lists information on drug assistance at their Web site (*http://www.cancer. org/docroot/MIT/content/MIT_3_2x_Prescription_Drug_ Assistance_Programs.asp*).

Generally, it is a good idea to keep receipts of all medical expenses for you, your spouse, and your children, as certain medical expenses may be tax deductible.

Throughout your treatment, track all of the financial costs that you have incurred as a result of this illness. Generally, it is a good idea to keep receipts of all medical expenses for you, your spouse, and your children, as certain medical expenses may be tax deductible. The IRS allows itemized medical deductions only to the extent they: (1) exceed 7.5% of the taxpayer's adjusted gross income and (2) are not compensated for by insurance or otherwise. Typically, expenses not covered by insurance are your annual deductible costs, co-pays (the fees you pay up front for specific services), and coinsurance (the part of the bill your insurance company doesn't cover). Other typical out-of-pocket expenses (e.g., prescription medications or the mileage for trips to appointments) may also be tax deductible. Unfortunately, the list of deductible medical expenses is too lengthy to discuss here, so please speak with your accountant or tax service when you are first diagnosed for information on what is tax deductible and what records you will have to keep.

Cancer of the esophagus is a rare type of cancer and not all facilities have experience taking care of patients with this diagnosis. If you have an HMO and do not have out-of-network coverage to see a specialist, work with your primary care doctor and the patient financial services department at the hospital where you want to be treated. They will be able to advocate on your behalf and write a letter of medical necessity as to why you need to see a specialist. Even with these efforts, your insurance company may still reject your claim. You may also call your insurance company directly and ask about out-of-network coverage to see a specialist. Keep track of who you speak with, the date of your conversation, and what the result was so that you will have documented records if needed.

Several tips to keep in mind regarding health insurance and medical bills are:

- Maintain the patient's current medical insurance policy—do not let it expire. Make sure to pay premiums on time. Patients who lose their jobs may be eligible for COBRA. COBRA allows you to keep the insurance for a limited time if the full premium is paid.

- Pre-certification is required for some medical procedures and treatments. Ask your insurance company if you need to obtain it or whether the healthcare provider will do it.

- Submit claims for all expenses as soon as you can. Keep records of bills that are paid and those that are not.

- Some insurance companies assign a case manager to patients with cancer. The case manager works with the patient and the hospital. If you feel this would be helpful, ask if a case manager can be assigned to the patient's case.

93. What problems may I face in getting life insurance after a cancer diagnosis?

Life insurance companies evaluate new policies based on personal information such as age, occupation, and health to measure your risk as a new policyholder. Unfortunately, having a pre-existing medical condition like cancer makes it unlikely that companies will cover you for life or extended care insurance. The longer you are away from diagnosis and treatment, the easier it will be to obtain coverage. Most companies will sell insurance to cancer survivors at normal rates if they are healthy for at least five years after diagnosis.

If you are employed or retired, check with your company to see if they have provided coverage as part of your current or retirement benefits. Some insurance companies specialize in providing insurance to people with medical conditions, and some even provide coverage specifically for individuals who have had cancer. The insurance company will want to know the specific type of cancer, dates of treatment, treatment methods, and if the cancer has spread to other sites. They may also require copies of your medical records and pathology reports. Look for a company that is rated A or better by A.M. Best (*http://www.ambest.com*) or Standard and Poor's (*http://www.standardandpoors.com*). Even with these specialized insurance companies, you may not be able to get coverage until you have been cancer free for at least two years, but they may be able to evaluate your case on an individual basis.

94. Should I take vitamin or herbal supplements? Are there alternative therapies recommended during treatment and recovery?

If you are eating a balanced diet, you should not need to take a vitamin supplement. However, during treatment for cancer of the esophagus, it may be difficult to eat a balanced diet. In this case, a multivitamin may be beneficial. Check with your doctor before starting a new vitamin or taking high doses of vitamins, because some may have adverse side effects with treatment. For instance, high doses of vitamin E may thin the blood and are not recommended prior to surgery or biopsies.

Herbs or botanicals are a type of dietary supplement that has a long history of use and of claimed health benefit. However, some herbs may cause health problems or may react with medications. Since herbs are not classified as drugs by the Food and Drug Administration, no federal standards exist and their actual content cannot be identified. In addition, many herbs and supplements claim to have benefits that have not been proven. A more scientific approach to the benefits of herbs is underway, and many clinical trials exist to test specific herbs and botanicals for benefits in the treatment of cancer. Check with your doctor or the Cancer Information Service (1-800-4-CANCER) for a list of clinical trials involving herbs or botanicals for cancer of the esophagus.

It is important to know that just because an herbal supplement is labeled "natural," this does not mean that it is safe and without any harmful side effects. Herbs are not benign and can act in a similar fashion to drugs, causing side effects and medical problems if taken incorrectly or at the wrong dose. For these reasons, it is important to consult your healthcare provider before using any supplements, especially if you are currently undergoing treatment. Your provider can discuss the known benefits and possible side effects of the supplement, or refer you to someone who can. Many hospitals and cancer centers now have staff who are knowledgeable about the use of herbs and supplements for cancer. These staff may be in the "Integrative Medicine" or "Complementary Medicine" department.

Herbs are not benign and can act in a similar fashion to drugs, causing side effects and medical problems if taken incorrectly or at the wrong dose.

For more information, contact the National Center for Complementary and Alternative Medicine (1-888-644-6226 or *http://www.nccam.nih.gov*). Memorial Sloan-Kettering Cancer Center has a Web site that lists herbs and botanicals, and provides objective information for health professionals and the public, including a clinical summary for each agent, adverse effects, and potential benefits or problems. You can access this site at *http://www.mskcc.org/aboutherbs*.

Bart's comment:

I have been taking supplements for 4 years, and I have found them to be doing the job. I would suggest that you talk to a doctor that focuses on supplements and your particular type of cancer and see what he recommends. It needs to make sense to you, as you need always to stay in control.

95. How do I cope with the fear of recurrence?

Recurrence

When a particular type of cancer has been treated but later returns either in the same type of tissues or in other areas of the body.

Cancer **recurrence** is the return of cancer after treatment and a period of time when no cancer was detectable. Having a fear of cancer recurrence is normal. If you feel afraid or anxious about your cancer recurring, it is important to realize that these feelings are normal and you should not criticize yourself for feeling this way. Try not to feel guilty. Accept how you feel, and realize that there are strategies that can help manage these feelings. One method is to express your feelings and talk about them with someone you trust. Joining a support group for survivors is a good way to discuss your feelings with others who are experiencing the same fears and anxieties. Keeping a journal is also a good way to explore your thoughts and feelings. It may also be helpful to discuss your fears with your physician. He or she may be able to discuss the normal recovery from cancer of the esophagus as well as symptoms to look out for. Being knowledgeable about what to expect can help to relieve unnecessary fears and worries. A good Web site to check is Cancer Net (*http://www.cancer.net*). This is the patient information Web site for the American Society of Clinical Oncology (ASCO) and provides oncologist-approved information on specific cancers and their treatment, clinical trials, coping, and side effects. The site includes information on cancer of the esophagus and is designed to help people with cancer make informed healthcare decisions.

As we've talked about in earlier questions, maintaining a healthy lifestyle by eating a well-balanced diet (Question 33), exercising regularly (Question 32), and getting enough sleep (Question 75) can help you cope with life after treatment for cancer. You'll feel better physically and emotionally, and will lower your chances of developing other health problems.

Coping strategies that helped as you went through treatment can also help with the fear of recurrence after treatment. If you've tried meditation, or joined a support group and found that to be beneficial, continue to do so after treatment has finished. If you've tried some strategies and are having difficulty coping with the fear of cancer recurrence, talk with your doctor about a referral to a social worker, psychologist, or other mental health professional. They will be able to help you focus on your feelings and work on ways to reduce anxiety and stress. It is important to remember that while you can't control whether your cancer is going to recur, you can control how much you let the fear of cancer recurrence impact your life.

If you are having difficulty coping with the fear of cancer recurrence, talk with your doctor about a referral to a social worker, psychologist, or other mental health professional.

Bart's comment:

Recurrence is always a concern, especially as my routine CAT scans and endoscopy check-ups come up throughout the year.

When cancer occurs, it quickly affects your control of what you plan to do in the future. There is always the stigma about planning for tomorrow when the uncertainty of being here weighs so heavily at times.

What has helped me is my ability to live each day to the fullest. I appreciate seeing a sunrise and stopping to smell the roses, and I thank God for that awareness. I appreciate the smaller things in life and this has enabled me to handle the recurrence issue. A positive self-image adds to the equation.

Someone 30 years ago gave me a banner that says, "Make where you are better because you are there." It is a great motto to live by and it has given me a positive outlook on life without losing the realism that we all have to die some-day. Whether cancer takes my life or another reason, taking the time now to live out this motto will serve me well when that time comes. At least I now think that way.

I have also developed another motto that says "God sits on my right shoulder and there is nothing that He and I together can't handle." Life is so much easier when it becomes Him and me working together.

PART SEVEN

If Treatment Fails: Advocacy and Support

Where does esophageal cancer usually spread?
What are the symptoms that indicate my
cancer has spread?

What happens if the cancer comes back?

My treatment doesn't seem to be working.
What should I do to prepare myself and
my family for the future?

More . . .

96. Where does esophageal cancer usually spread? What are the symptoms that indicate my cancer has spread?

Esophageal cancer can spread at or near the primary site (local recurrence), to the lymph nodes or tissues near the esophagus (regional recurrence), or to other organs or tissue far away from the original site (distance recurrence). Some common sites are the liver, abdominal cavity, and lymph nodes in the chest. You may have new symptoms such as difficulty swallowing or pain, but often the recurrence is found at a follow-up visit with your doctor prior to developing symptoms. It is important to follow up with your surgeon or oncologist after your treatment is completed. Follow-up tests such as CAT scans, endoscopy, and PET scans may identify recurrence early, and your physician can then determine the best treatment options.

Treatment for recurrent esophageal cancer depends on the site and extent of recurrence. Most often this treatment is considered palliative, and the goal is to relieve symptoms and improve quality of life. Surgery, chemotherapy, and radiation each may be used for treatment of recurrent esophageal cancer. Your surgeon and medical oncologist will discuss treatment options with you, including clinical trials.

97. What happens if the cancer comes back?

When cancer that has been thought to be cured or inactive returns, it is called a recurrence. This can occur weeks, months, or years after the initial diagnosis and treatment. When you were first diagnosed, treatment was aimed at destroying all the cancer cells in your body.

Sometimes, even with the best treatment, a small number of cancer cells are able to survive and may not be able to be detected until much later.

Depending on the site and extent of the recurrence, surgery, chemotherapy, radiation, or a combination of these may be the best treatment. Discuss with your doctor the treatment he or she recommends as well as the side effects and goals of that treatment.

This may be a difficult time that can lead to fear and anxiety as you begin treatment again. One way that may help to alleviate some of this fear is to learn as much as you can about what's happening and find support to help cope with your feelings and emotions. Discuss questions and fears you may have with your doctor, nurse, or other members of your treatment team. Write down your questions so that when you see your doctor, you will have a list of concerns in hand and won't forget to ask about something. It is also helpful to have a friend or relative go with you who can help you remember what was discussed.

It is also important at this time to take care of yourself mentally, physically, spiritually, and emotionally. As we've talked about in other questions, maintaining a healthy diet and getting moderate exercise can help you to feel better. Support groups are a good venue to discuss your feelings and emotions with others who may be experiencing the same things. Take time to do things that you enjoy, and spend time with people you enjoy.

Take time to do things that you enjoy, and spend time with people you enjoy.

When cancer returns, it may often lead to a sense of loss of control over your illness. It is important to know that this loss of control is not a loss of control over your future. You are able to control the way you approach each day.

Bart's comment:

From a patient's perspective, you are always in fear of hearing that the recent test you have taken has indicated a tumor and the signs are you have a recurrence. I experienced that in December 2003 when the doctors indicated a suspicious area on my CAT scan and indicated I should have a PET scan. When the PET scan came back positive, my surgeon ordered an endoscope with ultrasound with the idea of getting a tumor sample to see firsthand if I had a recurrence. When the gastroenterologist indicated he could not find a tumor to biopsy, you can imagine how I felt.

There was a period of time, though, between tests when I thought I had a recurrence, and my mind immediately went to how long do I have to live, will I see certain milestones in my life? I thought back on my life and recalled a banner that someone had given me many years ago—"Make where you are better because you are there"—and thought about those words and how important they were to me.

If I get a recurrence it does not mean a death sentence. With the drugs they have today and are developing for next year and the year after, I still can live a fruitful life and maintain good quality of life even with a recurrence. Sometimes we need to "stop and smell the roses" and think not of ourselves, but of our families and friends and the journey that we share.

I often think of the soldiers in their late teens or early twenties who have given their lives for us and how they were not given the opportunities that I have enjoyed, and how thankful I should be for having that special length of time.

There is another saying that I heard many years ago, and it stated "for all that is happening we thank you God and for all that there is to come." YES! I truly believe that there is nothing that God and I together can't handle, and it is that mainstay that has caused me to do the things I do, to help the people I help and feel great about each day of my life.

We never give-up, we never yield to the cancer, we simply fight with all our strength.

98. *My treatment doesn't seem to be working. What should I do to prepare myself and my family for the future?*

When treatment doesn't appear to be working, you may be faced with conflicting and difficult emotions. You may be concerned about loss of control over your illness, the impact of this on your family and friends, and the choices you must make regarding your care and treatment. It is important to live your life as well as you can. We have included some information in this question that we hope will help to ease your concerns.

At this time, you may think about death and dying. We all know that death is inevitable but we do not usually spend time thinking about it. When faced with thinking about death, we often change how we look at life, and this change in perspective can lead to a change in what we value and hold dear. Some patients describe this as a time when they realized the importance of living one day at a time. You may have considered these feelings when you were first diagnosed and your perspective may already have changed. It is important to keep in mind that there is no right or wrong way to feel. Consider your emotions and beliefs about life and death, and find meaning for yourself in these thoughts and beliefs.

Your family and friends can be important sources of emotional support to you throughout your illness. They need to understand as much as you do and will need time to consider your illness and their own feelings of anger, helplessness, fear, and concern. Let them know their support and love will help you cope during this difficult time. Honest and open communication at all times during your illness has tremendous benefits for you as well as your loved ones. Discussing concerns or feelings helps your loved ones understand what is important to you, and it may also help to alleviate some of the fears or anxieties you each are feeling. Keep in mind, however, that everyone handles difficult situations in their own way and may need time to cope with their feelings. Talking with a professional, either in a group or individual setting, is a good option for you and your family. Members of the clergy are also a good resource to discuss concerns.

Treatment options at the end of life are varied. As part of your treatment decisions, discuss your wishes with your doctor and medical team. Home care is a comfortable and realistic option for many patients. Home care can provide medications, nutritional supplements, physical therapy, and other complex nursing and medical procedures. Treatment in the home can ease the emotional and logistic burden of traveling to the hospital for care. A home health aide can assist with personal tasks such as bathing, dressing, and other personal care. The home healthcare team will work closely with you, your family, and your medical team to plan your care.

Hospice is another option for care at the end of life. The goal of hospice care is to maximize quality of life and minimize pain and is based on a team approach to care. Hospice can be provided at home, in the hospital, or at a separate facility. Hospice care not only focuses on the medical aspects of care, but also the emotional, spiritual, and social aspects. Your doctor, nurse, or social worker can discuss hospice care with you and provide information on services in your community.

In addition to your medical care, you may also want to plan for financial, legal, and emotional difficulties your family may face after your death. This is often very difficult, but planning for matters such as wills and debts now can eliminate problems your family may face later. You may want to consult with a social worker, lawyer, or your insurance company about questions related to financial or legal issues. Organizing documents and records can also help your family cope with the practical aspects of life. You may also consider planning a funeral or memorial service that conveys how you would like to be remembered. Discuss this with your family and clergy so that the service has a personal and special touch.

This is a difficult time for you and your family. Keeping lines of communication open and living each day to its fullest will allow you to cherish the good things all around you.

ADVOCACY

99. Where can I get more information?

It is always helpful to learn as much as you can about esophageal cancer and its treatment. Discuss questions or concerns with your doctor or nurse and take notes during your doctor visits. Information is available on the Internet and also at your public library or hospital library. We hope that this book has provided you with some helpful and meaningful information as you navigate the complex and often distressing course on which a diagnosis of esophageal cancer can lead you. We've also included some information on organizations that may be able to provide additional assistance.

Bart's comment:

Two Web sites that focus on patient experiences and are linked to individual patients who work through e-mail networks to develop questions and respond to those questions are http://www.eccafe.org *and* http://www.fightec.org.

100. What are some helpful Web sites and telephone numbers?

The Appendix that follows provides a list of many helpful Web sites, organizations, and other resources for patients and caregivers.

Appendix

American Cancer Society (ACS)
http://www.cancer.org
1599 Clifton Road, NE
Atlanta, GA 30329
Phone: 1-800-ACS-2345

American College of Gastroenterology
http://www.acg.gi.org
Web site includes a physician locator for gastroenterologists

Cancer Fund of America, Inc.
http://www.cfoa.org
2901 Breezewood Lane
Knoxville, TN 37921-1099
Phone: 865-938-5281

Cancer Treatment Centers of America
http://www.cancercenter.com
http://www.cancercenter.com/esophageal-cancer.cfm (esophageal specific)
Phone: 1-800-615-3055

Cancer*Care*, Inc.
http://www.cancercare.org
275 Seventh Avenue
New York, NY 10001
Phone: 1-800-813-HOPE

CancerNet

http://www.cancer.net
General Health
Phone: 1-888-651-3038
Fax: 571-366-9537

Mayo Clinic

http://www.mayoclinic.com
Good general health Web site for illnesses and medications

National Cancer Institute

http://www.cancer.gov
http://www.cancer.gov/cancerinfo/types/esophageal (esophageal specific)
Phone: 1-800-4-CANCER (Cancer Information Service)

National Coalition for Cancer Survivorship

http://www.canceradvocacy.org
1010 Wayne Avenue, Suite 770
Silver Spring, MD 20910
Phone: 1-888-650-9127
Phone: 1-877-NCCS-YES (to order the Cancer Survival Toolbox®)

OncoLink

http://www.oncolink.com
Use "quick search" to access esophageal cancer information.
http://www.oncolink.com/types/article.cfm?
    c=5&s=12&ss=769&id=9465 (esophageal specific)

WebMD

http://www.webmd.com
Good general health Web site

PRODUCTS

Back Be Nimble
http://www.backbenimble.com
Phone: 1-800-639-3746
Inflatable wedge for sleeping at 30°

GOVERNMENT AGENCIES THAT PROVIDE FINANCIAL ASSISTANCE

Hill-Burton Funds
http://www.hhs.gov/ocr
Federal assistance is available to those who are unable to pay, and
is provided by the Hill-Burton Act of Congress. Public and
nonprofit hospitals, nursing homes, and other medical facilities
may provide subsidized low-cost or no cost medical care to ful-
fill their community service obligation.
Phone: 1-800-368-1019
TDD: 1-800-537-7697

Social Security Administration (SSA)
http://www.ssa.gov
Office of Public Inquiries
Windsor Park Building
6401 Security Boulevard
Baltimore, MD 21235
Phone: 1-800-772-1213

Glossary

A

Adenocarcinoma: A malignant neoplasm of epithelial cells in a glandular or gland-like pattern.

Adjuvant therapy: Chemotherapy given after surgery to lessen the chances that cancer will recur.

Advance directives: Oral and written instructions containing your wishes for medical care if you are unable to speak for yourself; includes medical power of attorney and living will.

Anastomosis: A natural communication or connection, direct or indirect, between two blood vessels or other tubular structures; the surgical connection of severed organs to form a continuous channel.

Anastomotic leak: A condition in which the tissues have not healed completely from an esophagectomy and liquids or saliva leak into the chest cavity. To treat this condition, more time must be allowed for the tissues to heal completely or the patient undergoes further surgery.

Anemia: A condition in which the number of blood cells, amount of hemoglobin, and/or the volume of packed red blood cells is less than normal. Symptoms include pallor of the skin, shortness of breath, palpitations of the heart, and fatigue.

Aspiration: The inspiratory sucking into the airways of fluid or any foreign material, especially gastric contents.

B

Barium swallow: (also called upper GI series or esophagram) A type of radiology examination where a barium solution is drunk before the x-ray is taken to be able to visualize the esophagus, stomach, and duodenum.

Barrett's esophagus: A chronic ulceration of the lower esophagus from esophagitis or esophageal cancer; causes the normal lining to be replaced by cells similar to the stomach or intestine, which can tolerate the acid or bile without damage.

Benign tumor: A growth or mass of abnormal cells that does not invade or destroy adjacent normal tissue.

Biopsy: A process of removing tissue from a patient for diagnostic examination.

Bougie: A cylindrical instrument used for dilating constricted areas in tubular organs (such as the esophagus).

Brachytherapy: A type of radiation therapy where a source of irradiation (such as radioactive seeds) is implanted directly into or near the tumor permanently or for a specified time.

C

Cell: The smallest unit of living structure capable of independent existence. Cells are highly specialized in structure and function.

Chemoradiation: Chemotherapy used in combination with radiation therapy.

Chemotherapy: The use of drugs to kill cancer cells.

Computerized axial tomography (CAT) scan: A type of x-ray procedure that is painless and provides multiple pictures of the body in specific sections for diagnostic purposes.

Cytotoxic drugs: A type of pharmaceutical substance that is detrimental or destructive to cells.

D

Deep vein thrombosis: A blood clot that occurs in a deep-lying vein in the leg or pelvis.

Dietitian: A degreed professional who can develop a nutritious eating plan for an individual.

Dilatation: (also dilation) An outpatient treatment used to stretch the esophagus.

DNA (deoxyribonucleic acid): A type of nucleic acid found principally in the nuclei of animal and plant cells; considered to be the autoreproducing component of chromosomes and many viruses as well as the repository for hereditary characteristics.

Dumping syndrome: Post-surgical rapid gastric emptying; early dumping symptoms include nausea, vomiting, bloating, and diarrhea; late dumping symptoms include weakness, sweating, and dizziness.

Dysplasia: Abnormal development or growth of tissues, cells, or organs.

E

Endoscopic ultrasound or EUS: A type of endoscopy that uses sound waves for diagnostic purposes.

Endoscopy: (also called esophagoscopy or EGD) Examination of the interior of a canal or hollow viscus by means of a special instrument called an endoscope; the patient is sedated during the process.

Epidural catheter: A small tube placed under the skin through which medication can be administered to a patient, via a pump mechanism either at a low constant dose or when the patient presses a button, according to the physician's prescription.

Esophagectomy: The surgical removal of part or most of the diseased esophagus and part of the stomach, followed by the rebuilding of a new esophagus using tissue from the stomach or the small or large intestine.

Esophagitis: Irritation, inflammation, or damage of the esophagus caused by regurgitation of the acid gastric contents.

Esophagus: A portion of the digestive canal, shaped like a hollow tube, which connects the throat to the stomach. Controlled muscle contractions propel food and liquids into the stomach, and muscles at the stomach form a valve (esophageal sphincter) that prevents the stomach contents from coming back up into the esophagus.

External beam radiation therapy: A type of x-ray therapy that comes from a machine outside of the body, usually delivered daily in a specific series of treatments.

F

Feeding tube: A flexible tube passed through the nose and into the alimentary tract, through which liquid food is passed.

Fistula: An abnormal passage from a hollow organ to the body surface or from one organ to another.

Fundoplication: Suture of the fundus of the stomach completely or partly around the gastroesophageal junction to treat gastroesophageal reflux disease.

G

Gastroenterologist: A physician with special training in the function and disorders of the gastrointestinal system, including the stomach, intestines, and related organs of the gastrointestinal tract.

Gastroesophageal junction: Location where the stomach and esophagus meet, also known as the cardia.

Gastroesophageal reflux disease (GERD): A syndrome due to a structural or functional inability of the lower esophageal sphincter to prevent gastric juice from flooding back into the esophagus.

Gastrostomy tube (G-tube): A type of feeding tube that is inserted directly into the stomach; this procedure is done surgically and requires sedation.

H

H-2 blocker: Type of pharmaceutical drug used to treat GERD and Barrett's esophagus; examples include Tagamet, Pepcid, Zantac, and Axid.

Helicobacter pylori (H. pylori): A specific type of curved or spiral microorganism (bacterium) that colonizes on the surface of mucus-secreting columnar cells, secretes urease (which causes infection), and along with other dietary factors, leads to gastritis and peptic ulcer disease of the stomach. It may play a role in the development of dysplasia and metaplasia of gastric mucosa and distal gastric adenocarcinoma.

Hiatal hernia: A condition in which part of the stomach protrudes through the esophageal opening (esophageal hiatus) of the diaphragm.

I

Incentive spirometer: A device used to help the patient inhale and expand the lungs.

Intravenously: Injection or infusion of liquid, usually medication, directly through the skin into a vein.

J

Jejunostomy tube (J-tube): A type of feeding tube that is placed through the skin directly into the small bowel.

L

Laparoscopy: A type of surgery using a laparoscope, comprised of fiber optics and low-heat halogen bulbs that aid in the placement and use of other surgical tools. One or more tiny incisions enable precise incision, drainage, excision, cautery, ligation, suturing, and other surgical procedures.

Laser surgery: A surgical procedure using a device that concentrates high energies into an intense narrow beam of nondivergent monochromatic electromagnetic radiation; used in microsurgery, cauterization, and diagnostic purposes.

Lower esophageal sphincter (LES): A muscle located at the top of the stomach that opens and closes to keep stomach acid and bile from backing up into the esophagus.

M

Malignant tumor: A rapid growth of abnormal cells that replaces normal cells, invades other tissues and organs, may recur after attempted removal, and is likely to cause the death of the host if left inadequately treated.

Metaplasia: Transformation of an adult, fully-formed cell of one kind into an abnormal cell of another kind; an acquired condition (*see* Barrett's esophagus).

Metastasis: Transmission of cancer cells from an original site to one or more sites in the body.

Minimally invasive surgery: An operative procedure that results in the smallest possible incision or no incision at all; includes laparoscopic, laparoscopically-assisted, thoracoscopic, and endoscopic procedures.

Multimodality: The use of specialists in two or more disciplines to treat a specific disease; may include diagnostic testing, radiation, pharmaceuticals, or surgery.

N

Neoadjuvant therapy: Chemotherapy given before surgery to shrink or isolate the tumor.

O

Oncologist: A physician with specialized training in the science of the physical, chemical, and biological properties of neoplasms, including causation, pathogenesis, and treatment.

P

Palliation: Used to reduce the severity or relieve the pain of a disease or symptom, but is not a cure of the underlying condition.

Pathologist: A physician who practices, evaluates, and/or supervises diagnostic tests, using materials removed from living or dead patients, to determine the causes or nature of the disease change.

Patient-controlled analgesia (PCA): Medication for pain that the patient can self-administer by pressing a button; after surgery while in the hospital, a small tube is inserted so the medication can be pumped into a vein.

Percutaneous endoscopic gastrostomy (PEG-tube): A type of feeding tube for those with an intact gastrointestinal tract who are unable to consume sufficient calories to meet metabolic needs; an ~30 minute procedure that requires local anesthesia.

PET (positron emission tomography) scan: A type of scan that measures positron-emitting isotopes with short half-lives that the patient has ingested to assess metabolic and physiologic function rather than anatomic structure.

Photodynamic therapy (PDT): A type of surgery that uses an injection of photosensitizing drugs to highlight the cancerous cells and laser light through an endoscope to kill them.

Photosensitizing: A type of treatment where target cancer cells are illuminated by bioluminescent drugs.

Polyp: A general term used for any mass of tissue that bulges or projects outward or upward from the normal surface level; it is visible as a roundish structure growing from a mound-like base or a slender stalk.

Primary tumor: Location where the original tumor began.

Proton pump inhibitors: Type of pharmaceutical drug used to treat more complicated GERD (associated with bleeding or strictures); examples include Prilosec, Prevacid, Aciphex, Protonix, and Nexium.

Pulmonary embolism (PE): A blood clot that has broken away from the blood vessel wall and travels into the lung; a large clot can cause breathing problems and even death.

R

Radiologist: A physician specially trained in the diagnostic and/or therapeutic use of x-rays and radionuclides, radiation physics, and biology; also trained in diagnostic ultrasound and magnetic resonance imaging and applicable physics.

Recurrence: When a particular type of cancer has been treated but later returns either in the same type of tissues or in other areas of the body.

S

Simulation: A process in which specific areas on the cancer patient's body are marked, sometimes using computed tomography, in preparation for targeting the tumor(s) with radiation therapy.

Social worker: A degreed mental health professional who can provide counseling services to individuals and groups as well as help the patient network with community services and resources.

Squamous cell carcinoma: A malignant neoplasm derived from stratified squamous epithelium cells, such as those that line the esophagus.

Stent: A thread, rod, or catheter that is inserted into the cell wall of the esophagus to keep it open.

Stricture: A narrowing or tightening of a hollow structure.

T

Transhiatal esophagectomy: Surgical type of resection of the esophagus where the incision is made from the cervical section of the neck from above and up from the abdomen from below.

Transthoracic esophagogastrectomy: Surgical type of resection of the esophagus through a thoracotomy incision (breast bone to the umbilicus, plus another incision on the right side of the chest).

Tumor: Any swelling caused by an increased number of abnormal cells.

Index

Italicized page locators indicate a figure; tables are noted with a *t*.